Creating Beauty to Cure the Soul

Creating Beauty to Cure the Soul

Race and Psychology in the Shaping of

Aesthetic Surgery

Sander L. Gilman

DUKE UNIVERSITY PRESS   Durham / London 1998

© 1998 Duke University Press
All rights reserved
Printed in the United States of America on acid-free paper ♾
Typeset in Trump Mediaeval by Tseng Information Systems, Inc.
Library of Congress Cataloging-in-Publication Data
appear on the last printed page of this book.

This Book Is Dedicated to My Friends
in the Class of 1996–1997 at the Center for
Advanced Study in the Behavioral Sciences,
Stanford, California

Contents

Preface

The question of how our society strives to "make the body beautiful" is in one measure the story of how we turn to medicine to make us over and therefore to make us "happy" with our new faces and bodies. As one woman who had aesthetic surgery of the face to correct the result of an early operation for a tumor remarked, "The technology is there, the good clinics are safe, and I applaud women who think it's worth spending money on cosmetic surgery. It's money spent on themselves and their happiness."[1] The view is that a conflict between the desire to be seen as "beautiful" or "handsome" and the difficulties in achieving that end can lead to a general unhappiness with one's own body. The accepted wisdom is that if you understand your body as "ugly" you are bound to be "unhappy." The evident consequence of this view in modern society is not only that people attempt to change their bodies through diet or cosmetics or fashion, but that they turn more and more frequently to their surgeons in the pursuit of the "body beautiful" and the "happy soul."

The widespread acceptance of aesthetic surgery as a surgical specialty over the past century is self-evident. In 1992, 30,000 women in the United States had their breasts enlarged; 8,000 had them lifted and 40,000 had them reduced; 16,000 men and women had tummy tucks; 20,000 had chemical peels; 40,000 had collagen injections to fill out wrinkles; 50,000 had nose jobs; 50,000 had liposuction to remove fat; and 60,000 had eyelid corrections.[2] Ronald E. Iverson, president of the American Society of Plastic and Reconstructive Surgeons, presented in the spring of 1997 the 1996 statistics concerning the range and number of procedures available to "clients."[3] The procedures, however, were divided into two categories, aesthetic and reconstructive surgery. The top five most commonly performed aesthetic procedures were as follows:

1. Liposuction (109,353)
2. Breast Augmentation (87,704)
3. Eyelid Surgery (76,242)
4. Retin-A Treatment (74,382)
5. Face-lift (53,435)

The top five most often performed reconstructive procedures were as follows:

1. Tumor Removal (542,063)
2. Hand Surgery (153,581)
3. Other Reconstructive (146,470)
4. Lacerations (115,998)
5. Breast Reduction (57,679)

This distinction between aesthetic and reconstructive surgery is that of the medical profession. The line between the two is not easily drawn.

Each patient understood the procedure as having beneficial psychological effects: 59 percent said the surgery reduced their "self-consciousness"; 16.5 percent felt it improved their "social acceptance"; 14.7 percent felt it improved their professional chances; 5.6 percent found the change in their appearance "positive"; and 4 percent felt they received "increased admiration."[4] These statistics seem to indicate that the aesthetic surgery is understood to affect internal as well as external perceptions. This finding is underscored by many aesthetic surgeons' observations that, in most cases, a patient's self-representation of his or her "deformity" is far worse than it is in the surgeon's estimation.

It is important to note that the profession of aesthetic surgery recognizes that not only women have procedures. Already in 1992, 13 percent of aesthetic surgery patients were men. As of January 1997, men accounted for 33 percent of aesthetic procedures, an increase of 9 percent since 1988, according to the American Academy of Facial Plastic and Reconstructive Surgery.[5] The problem of trying to achieve the "body beautiful" and the "happy soul" through aesthetic surgery is thus not limited to women, in spite of the views of many feminist critics of aesthetic surgery. The pressure of the "beauty myth" on women is only half of the story—men too are often hyperaware of their appearance and strive to alter it. Here, too, the end of the story is the sense of happiness attributed to the gendered body, whether male or female. After all, it was a man, not a woman, who had the first modern "nose job"![6]

The problem of the unhappy body image is not only gendered, it also reflects a Western preoccupation with all "deviant" forms of the body, whether it is the sagging chin or the "Jewish" nose. It is also vital to note that it is not only the gym and the personal trainer to whom women and men turn for help in achieving their new bodies, but also the world of medicine and the surgeon. Both men and women seek medical help in reshaping their bodies (and the bodies of their male and female children). Their goal is their psychological not their physical "health."

Central to all of these desires is our understanding of how aesthetic surgery works or does not work. The claim that aesthetic surgery is a form of psychotherapy is the focus of this volume. Because of these presuppositions, I describe how the claims about the psychology of aesthetic surgery have been framed and how surgeons, clinical psychiatrists, and psychoanalysts have understood its efficacy or inefficacy. I also complicate the notion of the surgeon as psychotherapist by presenting the counterarguments. Some aesthetic surgeons warn that their beauty scalpels are not psychological tools as well. "We aren't a cure-all for a problem life," says Jim Pietraszek, who practices aesthetic surgery in La Jolla, California. "The ideal patient is someone who, in the aesthetic sense, is less than optimal, but who otherwise is well-adjusted."[7] This debate is an ongoing one, and it will be the purpose of this book to describe the claims as to what exactly does or does not "cure," especially when a "well-adjusted" patient is being treated. While aesthetic surgeons debate the nature of their profession, philosophers ask whether one can even speak of aesthetic surgery as medicine in the sense that it attempts to cure anything. The debates about the psychology of aesthetic surgery reflect the conflicted and often heated debate about the meanings associated with the aesthetic alteration of the body over the past one hundred years.

What you will read has had the benefit of discussions with friends and colleagues (sometimes the same people) at the Cornell Medical College, the University of Chicago, the Wellcome Institute for the History of Medicine (London), the University of Michigan, the Courtauld Institute (London), the School of Oriental Studies (London), the Center for Advanced Study in the Behavioral Sciences (Stanford, CA), and the National Library of Medicine (Bethesda, MD). My research assistants Rhoda Rosen, Veronika Fürchtner, and Katja Garloff were also of great help in putting this project on track.

This book draws on some of my earlier work, specifically discussions of aesthetic surgery in *The Jew's Body* (1991), *Freud, Race, and Gender* (1993), and *Health and Illness* (1995). It adds much to what may be found there and expands on the number of pieces in the cyber-jigsaw puzzle just a bit more.

This volume was completed while I was a fellow at the Center for Advanced Study in the Behavioral Sciences in Stanford, CA. I am grateful for financial support provided by the Andrew W. Mellon Foundation.

Part One

The Manufacture of Happiness

1. Reconstructing What?

From the beginning of the profession, reconstructive surgery, in restoring function, seems to lie at one end of a spectrum and aesthetic surgery, in improving appearance, at the other.[1] Even today, these two historically closely related forms of "plastic surgery" are perceived by many patients and physicians alike as antitheses, one being "serious" medicine, the other "frivolous" and, indeed, not really medicine at all. This distinction between "serious" reconstructive and "frivolous" aesthetic surgery is as old as the profession itself. One of the most knowledgeable aesthetic surgeons before World War I, Frederick Strange Kolle (1871–1929), was already puzzled by this distinction. He distinguished between the surgery of the nose applied to "deformities when caused by traumatism, the excision of neoplasms or destructive disease" and "such corrections [as] are made purely with the object of improving the nasal form when the deformity is either hereditary or the result of remote accident." He continued, however: "For some unaccountable reason [aesthetic surgery] has not met with the general favor the profession should grant it, yet the results obtained by such specialists as have undertaken this artistic branch of surgery have been all that could be desired, and have consequently added much to the comfort and happiness of the patient."[2] Kolle's distinction between reconstructive and aesthetic surgery is continued in a widely quoted aphorism by the New Zealand–born surgeon Harold Delf Gillies (1882–1960), who understood reconstructive surgery as "an attempt to return to normal; aesthetic surgery as an attempt to surpass the normal."[3] Gillies needed to provide a meaningful continuity between his reconstructive work during World War I and the postwar interest in aesthetic surgery. In doing so he stressed the continuity between two concepts of the "normal." The first is a reconstructive model, restoring function and a somewhat human visage that can "pass" as normal if the range and meaning of the trauma are understood. The second, that of aesthetic surgery, seeks to transcend the given and the normal. The arbitrariness of such a set of juxtapositions is clear: One culture's "normal" is another culture's ugly "deformity." What is visible in one culture as unaesthetic is (in)visible in another as a sign of "beauty." (In)visibility is the goal of all aesthetic procedures. Aesthetic procedures are intended to move an individual from being visible in one cohort to being a member of another cohort or collective, which is *so* visible that its visibility becomes defined as the "normal." The "normal" defines itself as invisible. A correlation to this is that not only is it important for the patient to become invisible, but (in his or her own estimation) the surgeon strives always to appear healthy and (in)visible.

The status of aesthetic surgery in the latter half of the nineteenth century and the early twentieth century was undermined because its stated goal was not to correct physical pathologies (such as a cleft palate) but to deal "with purely external characters for which the only guidance is the patient's whims," as Gustavo Sanvenero-Rosselli (1897–1974) claims in the major Italian textbook of rhinoplastic surgery, published in 1931.[4] The whims of the patient are the basis for the autonomy of the aesthetic surgical patient, who defines himself or herself as in need of surgery. Such negative views of patient autonomy seem to exist even today. One contemporary commentator on aesthetic surgery and ethics observes:

> Some plastic surgery, though, neither affirms nor conflicts with full human personhood. Such operations, not designed to repair a defect, seek to enhance already normal appearance. This "beauty surgery" . . . cannot be justified on medical grounds although it is morally unproblematic. "Non-medical" plastic surgery must be differentiated from the majority of procedures which are properly considered "medical." . . . Distinguishing medical from non-medical plastic surgery has ethical import: medical procedures, I maintain, provide preconditions for full personhood; non-medical procedures on the other hand may enhance physical beauty, fashionable appearance, etc. While the moral legitimacy of plastic surgery is judged by its

impact on the patient as person, the relative worth of these procedures is ascertained by considering the priority of the medical or non-medical values justifying them.[5]

Such views permeate some of the contemporary feminist discussions of aesthetic surgery as well. They relegate it not to the non-medical because it is based on the "false consciousness" of the individual patient and is therefore exploitative and destructive.[6] For these feminist critics, socialization of women into a "beauty" culture makes women believe themselves to be less than perfect. Aesthetic surgery becomes the means that the medical profession offers to achieve this false sense of belonging to the "normal" world of commodified beauty.

The premise of this book is that despite the firm conviction of the critics of aesthetic surgery, both from within and without the profession, what many see as the absolute border between "good" reconstructive and "bad" aesthetic surgery seems all too often to waver. In a recent overview of the psychological literature on aesthetic surgery, Hans-Peter Wengle defined aesthetic (cosmetic) surgery as dealing with the defects caused by "aging and developmental disproportions; plastic (reconstructive) surgery as that dealing with the deformities caused by disease, accident, malformation OR surgical interventions for aesthetic and functional reasons."[7] It is ironic that even errors in aesthetic surgery come within the purview of the reconstructive surgeon. The "official definition" of the American Society of Plastic and Reconstructive Surgeons (from 1987) does not evoke iatrogenic causes for aesthetic surgery: "Cosmetic surgery is performed to reshape normal structures of the body in order to improve the patient's appearance and self-esteem. Reconstructive surgery is performed on abnormal structures of the body, caused by congenital defects, developmental abnormalities, trauma, infection, tumors or disease. It is generally performed to improve function, but may also be done to approximate a normal appearance."[8] This definition was accepted by the American Medical Association in June 1989. According to such definitions, all procedures can be "aesthetic" even if they are "reconstructive," as they reconstruct or construct a Platonic ideal of the body. Most important, they postulate that the prime location for this "reconstruction" is the psyche.

Such a desire to place all surgery—reconstructive and aesthetic—into the same category is rooted in the social and professional stigma associated with being an aesthetic surgeon. (Here the corollary is also true: the desire to separate them is a sign of the stigma associated with the practice of aesthetic surgery.) In the popular imagination, one can see this operative in the 1991 Warner Bros.' film directed by Michael Caton-Jones, *Doc Hollywood* (based on a novel by Neil B. Schulman, MD[9]), in which Ben Stone (played by Michael J. Fox) is a brash, newly minted aesthetic surgeon whose trip West to open a lucrative practice in Beverly Hills takes a small-town detour. He ends up in the fictional town of Grady, South Carolina, Squash Capital of the South, where he "discovers" that "real" medical service can be more morally satisfying as a general practitioner than in his imagined role as an aesthetic surgeon to the stars.[10] The stigma of doing elective beauty procedures such as those ridiculed in *Doc Hollywood* is countered from the very beginning of this specialty by the views that the procedures have psychological effectiveness. Thus the physician's attitudes toward theories of the mind come to provide the rationale for aesthetic surgery.

Ronald E. Iverson commented that "the tremendous increase in the number of plastic surgery procedures shows both the need for reconstructive surgery and the desire for cosmetic surgery. It is interesting that the increase reflects the versatility of board-certified plastic surgeons who are trained to perform both complex microsurgery and the most current cosmetic procedures."[11] Here too the link between "reconstructive" and "aesthetic" procedures rehabilitates the aesthetic surgeon from the charge of pandering to the vanity of the patient.

Reconstructive surgeons need to make distinctions between "malformation," "deformation," and "disruptions." Such distinctions come to play an important categorizing (nosological) role in the modern treatment of "undesirable" forms of the body (dysmorphology). Deformations are seen as "anomalies that represent the normal response of tissue to unusual mechanical forces," while malformations "denote a primary problem in the morphogensis of a tissue"; disruptions are the "breakdown of a previously normal tissue."[12] These distinctions are ones that are clearly paralleled within aesthetic surgery. "Malformations" are aspects of the body with which the patient is born (such as the shape of the eyes or that of the nose), "deformations" come about during life (such as pendulous breasts), and "disruptions" can be represented in the breakdown of "normal" tissue or other features in the aging process. And yet this set of distinctions is rarely carried over into the debates about aesthetic surgery. To counter the stigma of "merely" pandering to the patient's vanity, aesthetic surgery has rooted itself not so much in an understanding of its role in "curing" the body as in the "curing" of the spirit.

It has been argued that reconstructive surgery prior to the nineteenth century and the introduction of antisepsis (no infection) and anesthesia (no pain) was undertaken only when it was a functional necessity. Surgeons operated only in cases such as in the rebuilding of birth defects or deformative injuries of the face. During the course of the nineteenth century, the idea that one could cure the illness of the character or of the psyche through the altering of the body is introduced within specific ideas of what is beautiful or ugly. This was seen as a natural extension of the role of the reconstructive surgeons, who repaired the psyche through the rebuilding of the body. They postulated a Platonic "normal" and "intact" body and read their ability to reconstruct that imagined intactness as simultaneously reconstituting "psychic health": "Facial deformities, detrimental to the person's looks, are the hardest to bear because they are fully exposed to the 'ruthless' scrutiny of all fellow men and make social contact hurtful, and often—unbearable . . . the earlier in life the appearance—or awareness—of a facial deformity, the deeper its impact on the mind of the afflicted. One only has to watch the behavior of children marked by a cleft palate or hare-lip."[13] As will become clear, such arguments are the core of the psychological theory of aesthetic surgery, but they are simultaneously part of the argument for reconstructive surgery. Curing the physically anomalous is curing the psychologically unhappy—this view provides the key to any understanding of the power of all surgery to alter the psyche. The "beautiful" becomes the "happy."

It is also evident that the aesthetic has a place in general surgery. Scarring has always been seen as an undesirable result of the surgical intervention in the body. As early as the Edwin Smith Surgical

Papyrus (3,000 B.C.E.) surgeons in Pharaonic Egypt were concerned about the aesthetic results of their interventions.[14] The Egyptians were careful to suture the edges of facial wounds. Even fractures of the nose bone were dealt with by forcing them into normal positions by means of "two plugs of linen, saturated with grease," that were inserted into the nostrils.[15] The Roman encyclopedist Aulus Cornelius Celsus (25 B.C.E.–50 C.E.) stressed the importance of the "beautiful" suture.[16] This approach can be traced through to the surgery of the late nineteenth and early twentieth centuries with plastic surgeons such as Erich Lexer (1867–1938) stressing the aesthetic ends of an operation as "an always more appreciated requirement of modern surgery."[17] Such a stress on the neatness and beauty of the closure was part of the image of the return to function following the operation. For the beautiful was a sign of the healthy, and in modernity the healthy becomes a sign of the happy. Central to this sense of happiness within the culture of medicine is the hope that the restoration of the body will not reveal any medical intervention. The scar reveals that the body has been ill or damaged, that the present body is not intact but "merely" restored. The scar shows the body not to be "natural" but inauthentic and constructed. It is intimation of mortality that vitiates any happiness as it indicates eventual dissolution and death.

If medicine is seen as the space to construct a healthy body unblemished by signs of mortality, aesthetic surgery becomes the exemplary site for this desire. Thom Jones, one of the brightest of the young American writers, powerfully evokes this theme in his tale of death and the aesthetic surgeon, "Ooh Baby Bay" (1995).[18] The Jaguar-driving Dr. Moses Galen (*nomen est omen:* Moses, the "divine hygienist," according to nineteenth-century texts, and Galen, the Roman surgeon) lives as a very successful aesthetic surgeon in Los Angeles. He had been a reconstructive surgeon in Africa, running "a cleft palate restoration clinic in Mogadishu in the early 70s" (121). Now he is being paged by the "hair transplant" he had done that morning because "the pressure bandages on his head were driving him nuts" (126). Galen's physician–girl friend in Los Angeles had been completely reconstructed by him: "her nose was too damn big, she asked if he could fix that. She was so pleased with the results that she had him do a little of this and that. Her beautifully high cheekbones had formerly been a little too shallow, the firm chin had been slightly recessive, but Moses fixed that. There had been crow's-feet and wrinkles and breasts far too small, but Galen took care of that, too" (129). He operates not so much to alter her body as to cure her anxiety.

Linda's anxiety is "What happened to my body? Where has all the time gone?" (129). Galen's own diabetic body also shows the passage and decay of time. His very role as an aesthetic surgeon is based on his own anxiety about decay and death: "There was no easy death. Human organisms were tough and it was hard for them to die. That's why Moses went into cosmetic surgery—so he didn't have to look at death, even though he had seen his share just the same. In and out of hospitals every day, you just couldn't escape the problem of your own mortality. Dead wasn't so bad; it was the damn dying" (144–45). The tale ends with Galen collapsing with a heart attack, hoping that Linda does not hear his cries so that he can die alone. Jones's story exemplifies one model of representing aesthetic surgery, as the means of denying death to insure happiness. This utopian hope is recognized as both desirable and impossible by the patients and the physicians alike, and yet it is part of the hidden desire that shapes all aesthetic surgery.

The image of an intact, healthy body is part of all surgery. And yet that sphere of surgery—aesthetic surgery—that expressly devotes itself to the reconstitution of the "happy psyche" through the constitution of an "intact," "ageless," "(in)visible," "beautiful" body has been highly stigmatized over the past century. Are such bodies real bodies or mere simulacra? The stigma of aesthetic surgery was felt not only on the part of the surgeon. The social response, in many cultures such as Brazil, was for "these patients to keep their surgery a secret, ashamed to confess their vanity to their friends and family."[19] Such secretiveness has multiple readings. Breast reduction can be read as a reconstructive or an aesthetic procedure. This was clear in the desire of the U.S. Food and Drug Administration in 1992 to ban as frivolous silicone implants for women who had not had mastectomies.[20] Such surgery is only "shameful" when it is understood as "aesthetic," camouflaging the body and enabling it to be understood as something that is "essentially" different from what it "is." The very boundary between reconstructive and aesthetic surgery is drawn differently in different cultures at different times, but it follows this guideline of the difference between the authentic and the inauthentic. It is clear in the histories of cosmetic surgery that aesthetic surgery was a "poor relation" (so Goumain and Izquierdo in 1957[21]) of reconstructive surgery because it was seen as providing an "inauthentic" body.

It is precisely this arena—the aesthetic rebuilding of the body—that is the most highly impacted by cultural definitions of authenticity. The explosion of the number of aesthetic procedures in the United States of (North) America and the United States of Brazil and the increase in aesthetic surgery in France, Germany, and the United Kingdom over the past decades are clear indicators that the border between an authentic and an inauthentic body is always changing. Aesthetic surgery is meeting with greater acceptance on the part of patients and physicians alike because the idea of the surgically altered body as inauthentic is becoming less and less compelling.

2. Psychic Pain

The decline of the stigma associated with aesthetic surgery is keyed to the change in the stigma associated with mental illness. Both illnesses were socially unacceptable as they reflected the pain and anguish of the "invisible" psyche rather than the concrete body.[1] The rise of a "Prozac Nation" in the past decade is built on the gradual acceptance of specific, socially acceptable therapies for mental illness, such as psychoanalysis and drug therapy, the history of which spans the same period of time as does the modern history of aesthetic surgery. It is no accident that Prozac has been nicknamed "instant sunshine, the happiness pill, cosmetic surgery for the brain."[2] In 1995 Peter A. Adamson, then the president of the American Academy of Facial Plastic and Reconstructive Surgery, stated, "survey numbers demonstrate that technological advances are making cosmetic and reconstructive procedures more accessible and desirable. Several factors, including the lessening of social stigma, refinements in procedures, and abbreviated recovery time, are leading to the younger generation embracing facial cosmetic surgery in large numbers."[3] This lessening of the stigma is not accidental, but parallel to the gradual acceptance of aesthetic surgery as a form of psychotherapy. It is no accident, since, as we shall see, psychotherapy and aesthetic surgery are closely intertwined in terms of their explanatory models.

There is a new public visibility of aesthetic surgery. Pick up any newspaper or magazine in the United States or the United Kingdom, look in the drawer of your hotel room night table in Rio de Janeiro (right next to the Gideon Bible), and you will find advertisements for aesthetic surgery. Early aesthetic surgeons were little different from other members of the medical profession and, like them, advertised their trade. But their advertising was understood by their peers as tasteless, as when J. Howard Crum (1888–c. 1970), who may well have developed the first face-lift techniques, performed nose jobs on three members of the same family "in the manner of vaudeville turns."[4] Five women and ten men in the audience fainted. In 1979 a federal court ruling allowed American aesthetic surgeons again to advertise their techniques.[5] Advertising reappeared and is now ubiquitous. Indeed, one's sense is that aesthetic surgery is the dominant subspecialty that now advertises in all media—including the Internet. This new public face is a sign of the weakening of the stigma on the part of the surgeon and the patient. No longer a "back alley" specialty, aesthetic surgery has become central to our cultural understanding of the body. It is thus as much of medical and popular culture as psychoanalysis. Even those psychotherapists who do not see themselves as psychoanalysts use psychoanalytic therapeutic techniques such as the "talking cure." Mass culture remains saturated with the basic premises of psychoanalysis. Western culture retains a psychoanalytically informed worldview.

The central assumption of aesthetic surgery is that if you understand your body as "bad" you are bound to be "unhappy." In examining the cultural fantasies about what arbitrarily differentiates the "good" body from the "bad" body, we can also see how these categories become the object of medical treatment. In modernity, being unhappy is identical with being sick, and if you are sick, you should be cured. The idea that you can cure the soul by altering the form of the body has become a commonplace in the twentieth century. The other side of the coin is that to cure specific somatic symptoms you need to "heal" the psyche.

Both of these views of the healing of the psyche, the first, that of aesthetic surgery and the second, of psychosomatic medicine and psychoanalysis, reflect developments within the medical and general cultures of the late nineteenth and early twentieth centuries. Edward Shorter in his histories of psychosomatic medicine has helped write part of that tale, and historians of psychoanalysis, such as myself, have contributed to an understanding of how the presumptions of psychoanalysis rest on a very specific, culturally formed understanding of the mind-body dichotomy.[6]

The analogy between the belief system of aesthetic surgery and the history and structure of psychoanalysis is even more complex. Sigmund Freud (1856–1939) recognized in the *Studies of Hysteria* (1895) that he had "often . . . compared cathartic psychotherapy with surgical intervention."[7] The model of surgical intervention on the nose that he proposed was originated by his friend Wilhelm Fliess, as we shall discuss later. These views of the psychotherapists of the 1890s present a powerful comment on the premises of aesthetic surgery as developed in the same decade. Freud commented that some cases of "hysterical" illnesses are indeed somatic in nature and he was "convinced that the patients would benefit if we were more often to hand over the treatment of these affections to the rhinological surgeons."[8] The basic premise of aesthetic surgery rests on the simple reversal of the psychosomatic model that underlies orthodox psychoanalysis. For the psychoanalyst, psychic "misery" is written on the body as physical symptoms; for the aesthetic surgeon, the "unhappiness" of the patient is the result of the physical nature of the body.

There are other striking similarities between the explanatory models of aesthetic surgery and psychoanalysis as well. In the history of psychoanalysis, like that of aesthetic surgery, it is the patients who approach the doctors with an account of their symptoms ("hysterical misery") and who also propose the form of the treatment. Thus the archetypal psychoanalytic patient, "Anna O." (Bertha Pappenheim [1859–1936]), informed Sigmund Freud's friend and colleague the Viennese neurologist Josef Breuer (1842–1925) in the early 1890s what was wrong with her (her physical symptoms) and how she wanted to be cured ("Chimney-sweeping," her term for the talking cure). This is quite unusual in the history of nineteenth-century medicine where most often it is the physician-scientist who describes the disease entity and then provides the cure. One can use as a model for such treatment the complex history of asylum psychiatry in the nineteenth century with its emphasis on the patient as object of treatment and the psychiatrist (alienist) as medical scientist supervising the patient's every action while defining and classifying the disease entity and its amelioration. It is against such a model of nineteenth-century medicine that both aesthetic surgery and psychoanalysis react.

Contemporary psychological theories of aesthetic surgery claim that the ability of the patient to tell a complete narrative is a predictor of positive outcome. Furthermore, that outcome is defined as the reconstitution of psychological health. Thus one of the major "signs" indicative of a negative psychological outcome in aesthetic surgery is the patient's inability to narrate what is wrong and to be specific in his or her desire for change.[9] This inability to narrate the account of one's illness and the specific means for its amelioration (the defining structure for the origins of aesthetic surgery and psychoanalysis) is a sign of psychological instability. In the world of aesthetic surgery, this instability is marked by the patient's unhappy repetition of surgical procedures. Hysterical patients, according to Freud in his 1905 account of the case of the hysterical patient "Dora," are unable to present a coherent account of their lives (unlike paretics who may manifest the same physical symptoms but can tell you their life story from beginning to end).[10]

One further parallel to the world of psychosomatic medicine should be noted. As with the discussion of the "praecox effect" in the study of schizophrenia during the 1950s, there seems to be an aesthetic "surgeon's intuitive response to the patient."[11] As an aesthetic surgeon, one simply knows a difficult or dangerous or unhappy patient when one sees one.[12] This learned response to the difficult patient places the surgeon in the position of the psychiatrist. The history of aesthetic surgery runs remarkably parallel to that of psychoanalysis as well as psychosomatic medicine.

Freud's understanding of health and illness was rooted in the concept of psychosomatic illness—illness that arises in the mind but has somatic as well as psychological symptoms. Building on the work of the German Romantic alienists, such as Johann Heinroth (1773–1843) and Karl Wilhelm Ideler (1765–1842), Freud evolved complex ideas regarding the relationship between illnesses of the mind and the state of the body. For him, the patient's body is what the patient's mind deems it to be.

Freud's ideas were not new even though they were innovative. The idea that the body and the mind were connected had antecedents in seventeenth- and eighteenth-century thought. The physiognomists, such as the eighteenth-century Swiss divine Johann Caspar Lavater (1741–1801), for example, believed that the character and the body were one. Even earlier, philosophical approaches in the seventeenth century, such as those of René Descartes (1596–1650) and Gottfried Wilhelm Leibniz (1646–1716), had provided models for the relationship between the mind and the body. Monistic theories, such as those of Descartes, saw the mind and body as one unit, with all aspects of one present automatically in the other. Leibniz's views were not quite as schematic, yet he believed that each aspect of the human being was necessarily linked in a "predisposed harmony" with other aspects. Such views attempted to bridge long-held dualistic views that mind and body were separate entities that bore little or no relationship one to the other.

The idea that body and mind were inexorably linked began to dominate the understanding of the body with the growing influence of the German Romantics at the beginning of the nineteenth century. The fascination with the "night side" of life, with the ill and the corrupt as well as with the psychologically unstable, became one of the hallmarks of Romantic fantasy. For the Romantics, the philosophical task was to define where precisely the interaction between mind and body took place. Carl Gustav Carus (1789–1869), in his book *Psyche* (1846), stated that the "unconscious was the key to the knowledge of the conscious life."[13] This view dominated the antimaterialist European medicine during the closing decades of the nineteenth century. Even materialists came to be influenced by this view. Jean Martin Charcot (1825–1893), the leading neurologist of nineteenth-century Paris, moved from an interest in the somatic results of brain lesions to an understanding of the physical nature of hysterical symptoms as the result of some hidden physical trauma. When Sigmund Freud went to study with Charcot in 1885–1886, it was to learn more about the problems of juvenile neurological problems. In Paris he was confronted with Charcot's hysterical patients and their physical symptoms and returned to Vienna convinced that the truth lay somewhere between Carus and Charcot. During the 1880s and 1890s Freud developed a complex theory of psychosomatic illness that located the illness process that produced physical symptoms, such as the *globus hystericus* (inability to speak), in the unconscious. His interest before 1895 focused on the conversion of psychological trauma (mind) into specifically related physical symptoms (body). Following 1896, his focus shifted to the fantasy of the patient, even though he never completely abandoned the possibility that "real" trauma could have an impact on the individual psyche.

Mental illness, illness of the psyche, could also be illness of the body. Followers of the "psychic" theory, such as Carus, assumed the primacy of the mind over the body. Such views ran counter to the views of materialist physicians of the time, the so-called "somaticists," such as Wilhelm Griesinger (1817–1868), who argued that "mind illness is brain illness," seeing the mind (and mental illness) as a product of the brain. All assumed that "mental illness" (always differently defined) was the core phenomenon that would prove their views. The psychic theorists developed the theories of psychosomatic illness; the materialists, the theories of somato-psychic illness. If one could show that the ill mind could create pathological effects in the body in the form of specific and defin-able symptoms or the other way around, one could move to treat one aspect of the monistic body-mind by treating the other. Mental illness was the means by which the physician could show the rela-tionship between the ill body and the ill mind. While Freud's own interest in psychosomatic illness lessened after 1895 with his aban-donment of trauma theory, he inspired a long line of psychoana-lysts from Georg Groddeck (1866–1934) to Alexander Mitscherlich (1908–) to examine the questions of the origins of physical illness in the psyche. Of all the psychoanalysts who wrote on psychoso-matic illness, none was more influential than the Berlin-Chicago psychoanalyst Franz Alexander (1891–1964). In Alexander's work one can see the refining of Freud's own views in Alexander's dis-tinction between conversion neurosis (hysteria) and psychosomatic illness. His most important work in this regard is his *The Medical Value of Psychoanalysis* (1936).[14]

Other approaches, such as the return of the fixed characters of physiognomy as the constitutional types of Ernst Kretschmer (1888–1964) in the 1920s, lead to work on a clinical theory of con-stitutions. Here the work of Friedrich Curtius (1896–) on the psy-chosomatic basis of colitis and asthma is typical of the application of a twentieth-century theory of types as a means of understanding how physical predisposition relates to mental and physiological states.[15] Of twentieth-century philosophers whose work served as an underpinning for much of the work on psychosomatics, none was more important than Victor von Weizsäcker (1886–1957). For von Weizsäcker, illnesses differ from individual patient to patient as each patient provides a different structure for his or her illness. Each illness is influenced by the psychic structure of the patient. These variations on the model of psychosomatic illness provide a wide range of positions for its possible interpretation.

The wide acceptance of the psychosomatic model is such that a range of seemingly contradictory views are built upon the idea of an absolute link between mind and body. The "somatopsychic" model that underlies the practice of aesthetic surgery lies in the reversal of the psychosomatic model. Here the view is that the "beautiful" body makes for a "healthy" psyche, that the "normal" body makes for a "normal" psyche. The rejection of a mind-body dualism in the twentieth century is total. Yet the problems of understanding how the "mind" and the "body" relate to each other remain constant. Indeed, the very continuation of a bipolar (if interconnected) model for "mind" and "body" suggests a continuing understanding of them as two different sites for illness and healing.

During this discussion, we have assumed the existence of a "body" and a "psyche" but they are far from being natural, unproblematic terms and require definition. In defining the body (and the psyche) my point of departure follows the view of Mary Douglas:

> The human body is always treated as an image of society and . . . there can be no natural way of considering the body that does not involve at the same time a social dimension. Interest in its apertures depends on the preoccupation with social exits and entrances, escape routes and invasions. If there is no concern to preserve social boundaries, I would not expect to find concern with bodily boundaries.[16]

Where and how a society defines the body and the psyche reflect how those in society define themselves. Thus there is a close relationship between the boundaries constructed between "patients" and "surgeons." These boundaries reflect other social and cultural boundaries in the society that begin to be articulated in the construction of both "body" and "psyche."

Octavio Paz, in his comments on American society (which actually are also comments on Western society) stressed the function of "hygienic taboos" such as those that underlie the psychology of aesthetic surgery. He noted that

> to comply with the precepts of hygiene means not only to obey physiological rules but also ethical principles: sobriety, moderation, reserve. The morals of separation inspire the hygienic rules. . . . hygiene is a social moral that has its basis in science. . . . The overlapping between science and Puritan morality permits, without recourse to direct coercion, the imposition of rules that condemn all singularities, all exceptions and deviations in a fashion no less categorical and implacable than any religious anathema. . . . Even though they wear the mask of science and hygiene, the function of the patterns of normality in the domain of eroticism is no different from the role of "healthy" cooking in relation to gastronomy. Both mean the removal or separation of that which is foreign, different, ambiguous, and impure.[17]

The notion of the body as a site of contestation, of purgation, of purification comes to link the body political and the aesthetic body as the focus of the surgeon's transformatory skills. Henry Schireson (1881–1949) prophesied in the 1930s that "plastic surgery with the esthetic as well as the reparative objective will be as commonplace in another five years as neatness and cleanliness are today."[18] For him, aesthetic surgery defines the border between the clean and the dirty. It is at this "border," "a vague and undetermined place created by the emotional residue of an unnatural boundary," according to the feminist writer Gloria Anzaldúa, that the marginal cases are to be found: "The squint-eyed, the perverse, the queer, the troublesome, the mongrel, the mulatto, the half-breed, the half-dead; in short, those who cross over, pass over, or go through the confines of the 'normal.'"[19] This is the slippery boundary that marks the world out of which aesthetic surgery developed and one that society uses to differentiate it from reconstructive surgery.

3. The Medicalization of Aesthetic Surgery

Modern aesthetic surgery began in Europe, specifically Germany, France, and the United Kingdom, and in the United States during the latter decades of the nineteenth century. From there it spread into every culture in the world, following paths of colonial and economic expansion and the domination of Western medical theory and practice. It followed the same path as the rise and spread of psychoanalysis. To examine the broader culture of aesthetic surgery we need to recreate the inner fantasies of such cultures as they constructed the medical reality of the "aesthetic body" and the "happy psyche" in Western Europe (Germany, France, Great Britain), North America (the United States and Canada), and somewhat later South America (Brazil and Argentina). To do so one must assume that there are shared cultural fantasies among nations with shared histories. In the West, the beautiful and the healthy (and the ugly and the diseased) are interchangeable concepts. Beauty surgery is understood as surgery to restore mental health, yet the understanding of what constitutes the "beautiful" and what constitutes the "healthy" shifts from culture to culture and from time to time. Only the relationship between the two remains constant. Making the body beautiful through aesthetic surgery is a means of restoring (mental) health. The power of the images of beauty and health in this tradition and its globalization has meant that models of aesthetic surgery with their origin in the European-American tradition have come to serve as the primary references for the development of aesthetic surgery in colonial as well as postcolonial cultures in South America, Africa, and Asia.

The globalization of both the procedures and the psychology of aesthetic surgery can be measured, for example, in the flourishing of aesthetic surgery by American- and European-trained surgeons in contemporary Argentina where "medical insurers say they have noticed an upsurge in claims for 'essential' nose jobs, while private clinics tout liposuction on the installment plan." This is seen as psychic improvement following the traditional model: "Argentines have long had a penchant for spending big on psychiatry and other forms of self-improvement. 'People have the feeling they can't control their own future; that working hard and being a good citizen won't get you anywhere,' suggests psychiatrist Marcelo Hernandez, 'That's why beauty has become the main value in the market.'"[1] The cultural concept of the "beautiful" includes standards of male as well as female beauty, but we shall see that the term "beautiful" is not a simple one—even within seemingly related and seemingly homogenous cultures.

To write the history of psychology within aesthetic surgery is to write an account of the aesthetic alteration of the mind and the body within the public sphere of medicine. It is their institutional as well as their cultural base that enables surgeons aesthetically to change the body. Other physical interventions into the body from hairweaving to tattooing and body piercing had been done throughout time and are in many ways related to aesthetic surgery. What changes in the late nineteenth century is the context in which these procedures are performed. Practices like tattooing have as their intent the creation of a cohort, all of whom bear identical physical form. These procedures are culturally ubiquitous but have a specifically modern form. In the Enlightenment, the desire to efface individual difference came to be part of the creation of a "public" face, and it slowly became the task of the physician and the surgeon to address this need to efface difference. As Richard Sennett notes, "Nowhere was the attempt to blot out the individual character of a person more evident than in the treatment of the face. Both men and women used face paint, either red or white, to conceal the natural color of the skin and any blemishes it might have."[2] What Sennett does not address is that the disguise of "blemishes" was the attempt to mask the real or imagined signs of syphilis, which were seen as written upon the face. Cosmetics becomes an adjunct of the treatment (or at least the disguise) of illness. It was the syphilitic who demanded that the missing nose or ulcerous lesion be masked in such a way as to render him or her (in)visible as one suffering from a stigmatizing illness. This demand was the basis for many of the technical innovations in aesthetic surgery from the sixteenth century to the nineteenth century. The expansion of the use of "cosmetics" is related to the creation of a cohort "seen" as acceptable. Aesthetic surgery, which has its modern origins in the Enlightenment, can be seen as the "modern" equivalent of such procedures. Indeed, the more common term "cosmetic surgery" has its origin in the late-nineteenth-century subspecialty of "medical cosmetics" in which the disguise of the syphilitic's symptoms was paramount.

The insightful cultural critic Lewis Mumford observed that "the structure of the human body, no less than its functions and its excreta, called forth early efforts at modification. The cutting or pasting together of the hair, the removal of the male foreskin, the piercing of the penis, the extirpation of the testicles, even the trepanning of the skull were among the many ingenious experiments man first made on himself."[3] Charles Darwin (1809–1882) had already claimed "that the same fashions in modifying the shape of the head, in ornamenting the hair, in painting, tattooing, perforating the nose, lips, or ears, in removing or filing teeth, etc., now prevail and have long prevailed in the most distant quarters of the earth. . . . They rather indicate the close similarity of the mind of man, to what ever race he may belong."[4] These were signs of the universality of the human being in the collective modification of the body as understood from the perspective of the Enlightenment. But Anthony Giddens has commented that "in [traditional cultures], where things stayed more or less the same from generation to generation on the level of the collectivity, the changed identity was clearly staked out—as when an individual moved from adolescence to adulthood."[5] This would be marked by the ritual alteration of the body. Giddens continues, "In the settings of modernity, by contrast, the altered self has to be explored and constructed as part of a reflexive process of connecting personal and social change." All of the changes in "traditional society" were seen as part of ritual and religion, dealing with the inner world of the spirit as well as with the world of the flesh. Unlike religious ritual, aesthetic surgery demands the putative autonomy of the individual inherent to the modern as the grounding for any choice as to how his or her body is to be altered. No such autonomy is possible within religious practice except where it internalizes secular norms that are not related to the body as such, as we shall see later in this book. Like body building, which also arises at the close of the nineteenth century, aesthetic surgery is a secular restructuring of body modification.[6] It arises, however, within that most radically secular of the institutions of modernity, the world of science and medicine.

Older, nonmedical procedures merge seamlessly into the practice of aesthetic surgery. The use of tattooing to create "the socalled 'Cupid's Bow' of the upper lip" before World War I is paralleled by the use of such tattooing for similar purposes (permanent eyeliner) at the end of the century.[7] And, indeed, in the 1990s the removal of tattoos through laser surgery has become a booming industry among aesthetic surgeons. Yet the meaning of "tattooing" seems to be quite different from the use of tattoos within religious ritual and its use within the autonomous culture of aesthetic surgery. That the medical meaning of tattooing parallels the rise of a culture of tattooing in the nineteenth and twentieth centuries is further proof of the potential for the parallel existence of similar practices within different social environments and with quite different meanings.

The movement of such actions as tattooing (often quite literally) into the public and cultural sphere of medicine gives them a quality of the "modern." The desire and need to transform the body, which are labeled as "universal," are present, but additional techniques in reforming the body evolve out of and become part of the culture of medicine. They move from signs of belief that mark and identify the body, to being seen as the means of masking the body, of making it (in)visible. In both cases they link the internal life of the individual to cultural institutions (ranging from circumcision societies to medical schools) devoted to altering the body.

Medicine, including aesthetic surgery, is also part of the general culture. In the general culture, too, ideas of how the psyche works are present. These images include assumptions about the relationship between the mind and the body. The idea of the cure of the psyche as central to the undertaking of aesthetic surgery postulates a "patient" with a "healthy" body but an "unhappy" soul. The very different definition of the patient as "healthy" within aesthetic surgery and the social awareness of this difference makes it imperative to examine how both surgeon and patient come to define themselves in terms of the understanding of what can be cured and by whom. How doctors and patients come to define themselves in aesthetic surgery is a large part of this story. The number of autobiographies of aesthetic surgeons provide a source for narratives about how physicians define and redefine their roles; often embedded in these and other more "scientific" narratives are first-hand patient accounts, clearly shaped as evidence by the surgeon.[8] Despite the fact that in many cases the patient's experience is recorded by the surgeon and therefore is subject to his screening, one can still learn how the roles of the surgeon as psychotherapist in this field have been carefully constructed over time. Their definition of their roles, but also of the nature of their own bodies— as objects of treatment and as professionals—come to define the very nature of aesthetic surgery. Parallel to the surgeon's definition of the parameters of aesthetic surgery, other forces in modern society were also staking out claims on the cure of the psyche and the dissolution of "unhappiness." Clinical psychiatry, psychoanalysis, psychology, psychotherapeutic social work, and even organized religion contest or support aesthetic surgery's claims. That is the substance of section 2 of this book. However, all such contestation is based on a seemingly "universal" set of assumptions concerning the basic relationship between "beauty" and "health," "ugliness" and "disease" that dominate modernity.

4. A Beautiful Body Is a Happy Mind

Aesthetic surgery is composed of those surgical interventions that claim that the acquisition of an idealized or imagined body type or physiognomy is a "cure" for "unhappiness." This is very different from Sigmund Freud's claims for psychoanalysis, which hopes, at best, to transform "your hysterical misery into common unhappiness."[1] Over the past decades people have turned more and more frequently to their surgeons rather than their psychotherapists in the pursuit of the "body beautiful" to achieve a "healthy psyche." Luis Majul, the author of a popular book on the rise of aesthetic surgery in Argentina, notes that the popularity of aesthetic surgery is the latest manifestation of a neurotic society that once looked to psychoanalysis as its path to happiness.[2] It has simply substituted one form of psychotherapy for another.

The relationship between the patient and the surgeon is a complicated and sometimes contradictory one. On the one hand, the patient hands over responsibility for his or her happiness to the surgeon. Rather than changing their bodies through diet or cosmetics or fashion, approaches that demand choices be made on the part of the individual, an ever growing number of people are turning this process over to those whom modern society empowers to deal with problems of physical and mental health, the physicians. Individual autonomy (with all of the limits on choice set by the world in which we live) seems to be replaced by the role of the dependent patient. On the other hand, the initial claim of aesthetic surgery as part of the world of the modern is that it provides a "real" choice for the patient; it is a sign of true patient autonomy. The patient defines the physical fault and how it makes him or her unhappy; the patient seeks out and may even determine the mode of therapy. Both of these claims are true. The most prestigious social institution in Western culture, modern medicine, has been involved in such "cures" of this sense of psychological discomfort with the body in an ever greater and more comprehensive manner since the last turn of the century. The role of the aesthetic surgeon, too, has evolved in terms of what one is permitted to understand as "cure." While patient autonomy in aesthetic surgery may well be greater than in other fields of medicine, it is still limited by the need to have the procedures performed by one who has been invested by the culture with the mantle of the surgeon.

Aesthetic surgeons operate on the body to heal the psyche. They perform operations designed to cure "unhappiness." Being unhappy is identified in Western culture with being sick. In our estimation only the physician can truly "cure" our spirits and our souls. This daunting task is no longer the purview of the cosmetician or the barber or the tailor. Even though Ovid (43 B.C.E.–17/18 C.E.), in his "Medicamenti faciei," spoke of makeup as a form of medication for the soul, today it is not at the spa or the gym or the hairdresser's that the most radical alterations of the body take place, but in the operating theater and the dentist's chair.[3] The ability (and the desire) to alter the body medically for aesthetic reasons is truly a development of medicine during the past one hundred years. It is of the same vintage as modern clinical psychiatry and psychoanalysis and springs from the same desire—to help heal the psyche. It is in this realm, the world of aesthetic surgery, where the most complicated questions about the relationship of the "beauty myth" to other categories of social and cultural organization must be asked.

The underlying assumptions about the definitions of aesthetic surgery have not radically altered since the mid–nineteenth century. One recent essay on the philosophy of aesthetic surgery by Christine E. Jones and Beulah D. Jones outlines these presuppositions as understood today.[4] They begin by defining the "fact" that aesthetic surgery deals with "patients of various ages, racial groups, men, women, gender dysphorics, and ethnic and cultural groups." The goal of the surgical procedures is to "provide the possibilities whereby to achieve the yearnings of the mind." The surgeon, however, is not a psychologist or psychotherapist, who wants to create mental health but rather an artist, whose "artistic ability to create," along with "the patient's willingness to be molded," assures the happiness of both. Happiness is defined as the ability "to offer external changes which are more compatible with the vision of the inner self."

Certainly one of the central questions of Western, "modern" society concerns autonomous individuals' being or becoming "happy." A front-page article on aesthetic surgery in the *Wall Street Journal* in January 1997 cited happiness as the major factor in the desire of people to borrow money to change their appearance: "Deborah Gross knows all about the demand that Mr. [Michael] Smartt [of Jayhawk Acceptance Corp.] is tapping. The 26-year-old secretary in Fort Worth, Texas, says she has wanted to enlarge her breasts for years. 'I've never been completely happy with my body,' she says. 'I just didn't feel right in a bikini.'"[5] This is a trope long associated with aesthetic surgery. On a program concerning the controversy over silicone breast implants on *The MacNeil/Lehrer NewsHour* (November 13, 1991) one commentator observed: "Over 2 million American women have had the same surgery this woman in Chicago had this morning. Unhappy with her breast size, she wanted breast implants to make her breasts larger." Such truisms are spoken, for example, by the Wonderbra spokesman Genevieve Nikolopulos, who commented to a reporter that "women who have breast implants tend to be extremely unhappy with their body in general."[6] Or, as a correspondent in China begins an article on aesthetic surgery: "Okay, Fred, you're horribly mean to everyone. Happy? A businessman from Australia is offering some remarkable cosmetic surgery in Hong Kong. Without going into detail (this is a family newspaper), he says he can increase the length and girth of a popular appendage by three centimeters."[7] Breast implants and penile surgery all provide patients who chose to have such procedures with a path to happiness.

Happiness is also the goal of the surgeon, as Dr. Leonard Levine, a Florida aesthetic surgeon notes: "'Mine is a happy specialty,' he says of his practice, 75% of which is cosmetic surgery on healthy people. 'I'm stamping out ugliness, whether it's a scar on a face, a nose someone is self-conscious about, or a body part out of proportion. It's all about symmetry.'"[8] It is symmetry of the mind and body, not only of the parts of the body themselves: "The pure aesthetic considerations of the surgeon . . . will not achieve the desired result, namely to correct the patient's inability to accept how he sees himself, if they fail to correlate with the needs of the patient and the attitudes of his daily contacts."[9] Indeed, one standard study of the psychology of aesthetic surgery states that the "creed of a cosmetic surgeon [is] 'If you're happy, I'm happy.'"[10] And it continues: "If the patient expresses pleasure in the operative result then the operation is a success that should not be tampered with no matter what the surgeon thinks." The patient's autonomy is definitive in deciding the success of the procedure in creating "happiness." Even the surgeon's happiness becomes dependent on the happiness of the patient.

Happiness in this form is a "peculiarly modern, Western idea," as the sociologist Richard Sennett comments.[11] Thomas Jefferson did include the pursuit of "happiness" in his Enlightenment list of the ideal goals of the autonomous citizen. By the late nineteenth century the belief that "unhappiness" is an illness that can be "cured" by the surgeon seems to be an entrenched belief. Indeed it was the Portland, Oregon, "beauty" surgeon Adalbert G. Bettman (1883–?) who wrote in 1929 that aesthetic surgery "has been perfected to such a degree that it is now available for the improvement of the patient's mental well-being, their pursuit of happiness."[12] But what exactly is the happiness to be pursued?

"Happiness" was the goal of much ethical philosophy from the ancient world to the Enlightenment.[13] "Eudaimonia," the term that Aristotle uses, is for him that goal that all men are deemed *collectively* to pursue. Even though what constitutes "happiness" differs from system to system even within the ancient world, it remains a quality of the collective. Aristippus the Cyrenaic means only "pleasant feelings" when he evokes "happiness," while Ariston the Stoic sees "happiness" solely in devotion to virtue. Hegesias states flatly that "happiness" is both "entirely impossible" and "nonexistent" since all pleasure is transitory. Yet all see happiness as an attribute of the collectivity, rather than that of the individual.

The Enlightenment marks the break between the idea of a *collective* morality and "happiness." The "pursuit of happiness" is no longer a collective goal but an *individual* desire. The individual must have the ability to pursue his or her (legal and moral) happiness whatever the overall goals of the society. "Happiness" is the goal of the individual within the Enlightened definition of autonomy. Human autonomy defines and is defined by "happiness" as one of its primary goals.

By the nineteenth century and the rise of aesthetic surgery the utilitarian notion of happiness stressed the autonomy of the individual, as found in chapter 2 of *Utilitarianism* (1863) by John Stuart Mill (1806–1873). In what becomes a commonplace, Mill writes that "actions are right in proportion as they tend to promote happiness; wrong as they tend to produce the reverse of happiness."[14] And Mill focuses on the happiness of the individual as his highest good. This is a sort of post-Kantian ideal categorical imperative of happiness. A right action is defined by individual desire limited by its impact on others. This becomes the ethical underpinning for all of the later discussions of aesthetic surgery in the latter half of the nineteenth century.

In his emphasis on the right of the *individual* to pursue happiness, Mill evokes Jeremy Bentham (1748–1832), who stresses in *Principles of Morals and Legislation* (1781) that "happiness" is to be regarded in relationship to the community or "if a particular individual, then the happiness of that individual."[15] This view certainly reaches its apogee in the 1911 definition of "happiness" by Ambrose Bierce (1842–c. 1914) as "an agreeable sensation arising from contemplating the misery of another."[16] No communitarian sensibility remains here at all; all "happiness" is summarized in an ironic condemnation of an individual subjectivity. The "happiness" seen as the goal of aesthetic surgery is equally contested and confused. It remains the uncontested goal of the aesthetic surgeon, and yet its meaning remains diffuse and historically determined. Certainly conservative thinkers such as the philosopher-physician Leon Kass condemn "happiness [as] a false goal for medicine. By gerrymandering the definition of health to comprise a 'state of complete physical, mental, and social well-being,' the World Health Organization has in effect maintained that happiness is the doctor's business (even if he needs outside partners in this enterprise)."[17] Kass goes on to condemn psychotropic drugs and the "claim that the alteration of human nature . . . is the proper end for medicine" (161). The goal of individual autonomy is, however, seen as vital in such discussions, even if only on the part of the physician. "Happiness" of the individual as defined by the individual is the goal of aesthetic surgery. And as such it is one with the claims of post-Enlightenment "modernity."

But were such aesthetic alterations of the body a "restoration" of an ideal, "happy" type, or were they a correction to or a masking of an inherently unhealthy type to make that person only appear healthy and happy? Is Ambrose Bierce really right? Are we happy only when we know our own value (and that of our body) as contrasted with the inauthentic, invalid body of the Other? As early as classical Greece (in the pseudo-Aristotelian physiognomy), it was observed that "permanent bodily signs will indicate permanent mental qualities, what about those that come and go? How can they be true signs if the mental character does not also come and go?"[18] Central to the project of aesthetic surgery is the assumption that all physical changes are changes to the psyche and that the restoration to a Platonic ideal of beauty and happiness (through the invisibility of the subject) is possible. And here the inherent contradiction of the Enlightenment promise of individual transformation is present. If you assume a system in which outward appearance and inner life are bound in an absolute or contingent manner, aesthetic surgery can be only "superficial" and therefore not medical at all. In such cases it is cosmetic rather that somatopsychic surgery. This comes to be the problem for aesthetic surgeons in the course of the establishment of their specialty, and it is the need to document the psychological "happiness" of the patient as the proof of the efficacy of the surgical intervention that is necessary.

"I will follow that system or regimen which, according to my ability and judgment, I consider for the benefit of my patients, and abstain from whatever is deleterious and mischievous," states the Hippocratic oath taken by physicians over the past hundred years. In other words, the very idea of modern medicine remains inextricably tied to "cure." Is aesthetic surgery "deleterious and mischievous" because it operates on a "healthy" body? Joseph M. Rosen, an aesthetic and reconstructive surgeon at the Dartmouth-Hitchcock Medical Center in Lebanon, New Hampshire, who imagines his specialty creating the masters and monsters of the next millennium, gleefully noted, "We actually operate on people who are normal. It's amazing that we're allowed to do that, the idea that we can get a permit to operate on someone who is totally normal is an unbelievable privilege. In a way it's the ultimate surgery."[19] Aesthetic surgery comes to understand itself not only as not doing harm in altering the body but as improving the psyche, and therefore, fulfilling the Hippocratic obligation of the physician to do no harm.

The idea of "unhappiness" is closely tied to that of a psyche impacted by the social or cultural definition of the body. It is shaped by the notion of somatic and mental pain that haunts this tale, and it is no accident that these shifts take place in the latter half of the nineteenth century. As the cultural critic Elaine Scarry has remarked, "At particular moments when there is within a society a crisis of belief—that is, when some central idea or ideology or cultural construct has ceased to elicit a population's belief either because it is manifestly fictitious or because it has for some reason been divested of ordinary forms of transubstantiation—the sheer material factualness of the human body will be borrowed to lend that cultural construct the aura of 'realness' and 'certainty.' "[20] It is this reality and certainty that are ascribed to the imagined as well as to the real body that is operated upon by the aesthetic surgeon. These bodies possess the potential for change and for the pursuit of happiness, but such transmutations hold within them the notion that no such transubstantiation is truly possible, that the pursuit of happiness is a chimera.

The aesthetic surgeon constructs the (in)visible, the erotic, and the sensual as opposed to the visible, the ugly, the corrupt. It is the promise to reconstruct the psyche to blot out the image of disease, to restore the body, not simply functionally, but also aesthetically. But is this truly possible? In this worldview the idea of the aesthetic is intimately tied to those categories, as Paz has argued, that are labeled as unhealthy and corrupt. The measure of this attractiveness lies in the sense that the individual "likes" his or her body. You hate what the society hates. If your body (and therefore your psyche) is marked as different, diseased and foul, you internalize it as unhealthy and you become "unhappy" with it. Thus the mark of the healthy body is the happy soul—*mens sana in corpore sano*—or perhaps, closer to the reality, the mark of the unhealthy body is the sick soul—*mens non sana in corpore insano.*

5. The Phantom of the Opéra's Nose

The unhealthy soul is mirrored in (or caused by) the unhappy face. No more unhappy a psyche can be imagined in modern culture at the very beginning of our modern fascination with aesthetic surgery than that of the protagonist in the novel *The Phantom of the Opéra* (1911) by Gaston Leroux (1868–1927). Here the Phantom's "mask" is truly only a mask and the image of the diseased gives the reader access to the popular fears surrounding the erotic. "The Opéra ghost really existed," or so Leroux claimed at the very beginning of his novel.[1] In a true sense the Opéra ghost really did exist— at least the horror that the hidden face of the Phantom evoked was quite real to Leroux's readers and to readers ever since.

What was it about the potential sight of Erik, the Phantom of the Opéra, that so terrified (and fascinated) Leroux's audience (and us)? As readers we are given glimpses of the ghost's face through the eyes of the members of the Opéra very early in the book, and they are frightening. The Phantom's masked face had "eyes . . . so deep that you can hardly see the fixed pupils. You just see two big black holes, as in a dead man's skull. His skin, which is stretched across his bones like a drumhead, is not white, but a nasty yellow. His nose is so little worth talking about that you can't see it side-face; and the absence of that nose is a horrible thing to look at." This nose is so tiny that it seems to be missing. His nose seems to be the locus of the horror felt by the viewers as well as by the ghost himself. The Phantom often sports a "long, thin, and transparent" nose that is evidently "a false nose" (30): "When he went out in the streets or ventured to show himself in public, he wore a pasteboard nose, with a mustache attached to it, instead of his own horrible hole of a nose. This did not quite take away his corpse-like air, but it made him almost, I say almost, endurable to look at" (207). His missing nose led him to hate those with "real noses" and gave his face the aura of a death's head (227). Indeed, the ghost "smelt of death" (126). He felt himself as "built up of death from head to foot" with "his terrible dead flesh" (129).

Indeed, evoking the physiognomy of syphilis was a commonplace in the Enlightenment as a means of discarding all notions of this world's being the "best of all possible worlds." Syphilis marked the face of the naive and the innocent as well as the lecher and hypocrite. Voltaire (1694–1778) too had his Candide discover his teacher, the incurably optimistic philosopher Dr. Pangloss, "all covered with scabs, his eyes sunk in his head, the end of his nose eaten off, his mouth drawn on one side, his teeth as black as a cloak, snuffling and coughing most violently, and every time he attempted to spit out dropped a tooth." His is the last face in a long litany of diseased physiognomies in the literature of the Enlightenment. The cause of his dilemma was "Pacquette, that pretty wench, who waited on our noble Baroness; in her arms I tasted the pleasures of Paradise, which produced these Hell torments with which you see me devoured. She was infected with an ailment, and perhaps has since died of it; she received this present of a learned Franciscan, who derived it from the fountainhead; he was indebted for it to an old countess, who had it of a captain of horse, who had it of a marchioness, who had it of a page, the page had it of a Jesuit, who, during his novitiate, had it in a direct line from one of the fellow adventurers of Christopher Columbus; for my part I shall give it to nobody, I am a dying man."[2] The face of syphilis is the face of death, a death with a long history.

The image of the Phantom, his unrequited love of the soprano Christine Daaé, the singer whom he tutors and eventually abandons, is built about the horrid aspect of his face. What does the mask conceal? We see his face very early on in the novel and its very physiognomy reveals what is at the center of Erik's horror—branded on his physiognomy are the scars of congenital syphilis. The missing nose, the fixed pupils, the stench of rotting flesh are all (at least in the popular mind of the turn of the century) indicators of the social disease that marks Erik. His own horror at his obsessive love of Christine Daaé, his desire for consummation of his love and his rejection of it, is rooted in his repugnance toward his own body. His artificial nose is a sign that contemporary readers would understand as a visible mark of his disease. Erik's tragedy is that his illness was not of his making. He was born malformed, "his ugliness a subject of horror and terror to his parents" (261). Their horror pointed to the social stigmatization of their own sexuality, visible now for everyone to see in the deformity of their son.

The erotic and the reproductive are linked at the turn of the century through the concept of hereditary syphilis. The tiny nose represents a castration, not merely as an attenuated fin de siècle metaphor, but as a real action: not only social castration, but the demand that infected people not reproduce. Erik is the product of individuals whose sexuality was polluted and whose pollution is proven by the deformity of their child. It is the male who is represented here as infected, not the female who is seen as infecting. This is the case again in the sickly boy-child of the infected prostitute Nana in the novel named for her by Emile Zola (1840–1902). The child's death is obliquely recorded early in Zola's novel of 1880. Such individuals cannot be erotically attractive, since to be attractive would be a sign of the potential and even the desirability of reproduction. The hidden sexual pollution of the parents inscribes itself as deformity on the body of the children, who should be the moral force for the future.

The fright generated by the masked phantom of the Opéra, the dread that captured audiences from the 1925 silent film with Lon Chaney to Andrew Lloyd Weber's musical of the 1980s is the horror of what lay under the mask. What does Erik look like? What is striking is that the question that should immediately occur to the contemporary viewer now or at the turn of the century is why did Erik not have his face rebuilt? Why is it, that at the very moment when aesthetic surgery was being legitimized, at the moment when the reconstituting of the body became an adjunct to the healing of the mind, a novel about facial deformity came to capture the attention of all of Europe? Leroux wrote his novel exactly at that moment in history when the possibility of aesthetic surgery on the body and the psyche was becoming widely acknowledged. And certainly the reality of reconstructive surgery was already part of the medical (as well as popular) consciousness. It is not as if there was not a French literary parallel for the use of aesthetic surgery as a means of intervening in the moral dilemma of the lost nose. One of the most popular novels of Edmond About (1828–1885), *Le Nez d'un notaire* (1863), dealt with the dilemma of the title figure's lost nose and his unhappy search for someone to provide a source for his new one.[3] This text was in print well into the 1930s. About's rejection of the possibility of aesthetic surgery during the age in which aesthetic surgery becomes commonplace echoes his conservative account of the impossibility for physical and moral transformation.

The Phantom of the Opéra, however, is not a novel of the age of aesthetic surgery, but one of the previous age as seen from the standpoint of the modern. Leroux writes the novel as an historical one—looking back at the 1880s and the reign of the Opéra ghost—at an age in which such surgery was still marked by the stigma of syphilis. All lost noses, according to the common wisdom of the nineteenth century, the age of syphilophobia, were signs of sin. The Berlin reconstructive surgeon Johann Friedrich Dieffenbach (1792–1847) wrote in 1834 that "a man without a nose [arouses] horror and loathing and people are apt to regard the deformity as a just punishment for his sins. This division of disease, or even more their consequences, into blameworthy and blameless is strange. . . . As if all people with noses were always guiltless! No one ever asks whether the nose was lost because a beam fell on it, or whether it was destroyed by scrofula or syphilis."[4] As with About's character (who supposedly lost his nose in a duel), morality demands that the body be permanently marked even unto the seventh generation. In this fictive world, the ability to repair the moral damage caused by the parents is an impossibility. It is as impossible as the ability of the French to recuperate the infections caused by the demimonde that led (according to Zola's *Nana*) to the defeat of the French army by the Germans at Sedan. Erik, with all of his technological weapons and his colonial experience, cannot reproduce himself, for he will simply pass on the curse written on his face to all subsequent generations. No "mask" can hide this, even the mask of surgery. *The Phantom of the Opéra* is thus a novel in which the promises of the "happiness" of "modern" life have not yet been fulfilled.

The technology of destruction was in place. Erik could threaten to demolish the Paris Opéra with his kegs of black powder, but the technology of aesthetic reconstruction was not yet popularly accepted. The tensions about the promise of a new life in a new age and the destructive forces of the old century play themselves out in the physiognomy of the Opéra ghost and his potential for redemption. Like Nana and her child, he remains the unreconstructed symbol of the pollution present beneath the mask of middle-class French respectability. It is not divine redemption that is the focus of this work, but the impossibility of any human intervention to truly redeem the protagonist. In the 1880s reconstructive surgery could have created a new nose for Erik but even his reconstructed (and thus scarred) visage would have evoked a specific world of horror and disease.

Erik is not John Merrick ("The Elephant Man") (c. 1862/3–1890) whose deformities were the subject of both Victorian curiosity and charity.[5] Merrick's deformed face evoked pity; Erik's face, the face of the syphilitic, evoked the horror of contagion. Merrick became deformed; Erik's deformity was evident at birth. Merrick's illness too could have been altered by reconstructive procedures, but he chose not to have these done. They would not have eliminated, but only ameliorated his facial deformity.

By the time Leroux came to write his novel in 1911, Theodor Billroth (1829–1894), the famed nineteenth-century Viennese surgeon, often carried out "plastic operations with artistic ability to correct defects of beauty [Schönheitsgebrechen] . . . one could see his joy when he was able to successfully improve the appearance of [verschönern] a damaged person, so that that person was no longer the object of pity or horror."[6] The description of Billroth's Viennese patients was articulated in a language parallel to that which described the effect that Erik's physiognomy had upon his contemporaries. It was "pity and horror," the classical description of the roots of tragedy. Merrick is always represented as a positive figure; Erik, as a flawed, negative one. Ideally, surgery might have helped the former, but would not have changed the latter's soul.

It is no wonder that the putative etiology of the Phantom of the Opéra's deformity shifts over time. The 1925 American film, directed by Rupert Julien (1889–1943) and starring Lon Chaney (1883–1930) as the Phantom, evokes Leroux's etiology in the "pity and horror" felt by the audience in seeing the Phantom's visage.

Chaney adapts the standard physiognomy of hereditary syphilis for his makeup, which represents Erik's missing nose as a sign of the diseased soul. By the time that Arthur Lubin (1901–) made his 1943 film with Claude Rains (1889–1967) as Erik, the rationale for his disfigurement is quite different. He had been scarred by acid thrown at him by the engraver of his opera, who he believed wished to betray him. His face is scarred, he is not born disfigured. It remains a sign of an unstable (and certainly very unhappy) psyche.

If we sought a medical parallel to this moral dilemma as presented by Leroux, we would find it in the case of the princess and her sunken nose. Is Erik the ugly princess or Amy, the beautiful baby with her saddle nose? The missing nose of the Phantom demanded attention as a sign of the decay of inherited syphilis. The Phantom is a tragic character, for his nose can be replaced (at least in 1911) but his wound is one that demands attention to its cause. His "sin" is the sin of the parents, and that cannot be erased through a surgical procedure. It is not having been dropped on one's nose or even the misuse of the forceps at delivery. The problem of the morality associated with the ugliness understood of the missing nose is clear. It is a sign of the corruption of the parents.

The discomfort of the saddle nose is the discomfort of being identified as different, as pathological, as corrupt (and corrupting). The reconstituted nose, at least as proposed by all of the surgeons from Dieffenbach on, left its mark on the face through some type of scarring. If a forehead flap graft was used it was the mark on the forehead; if the septum was operated on through incisions in the skin, scars remained on the face. What such patients demanded was a total invisibility of the changes to their appearance. Their demand was a nose like everyone else's nose and thus the development of intranasal intervention for noses that were seen as "too small."

One should not imagine that the nose of the Phantom has simply vanished from popular representations of difference. With the "disappearance" of syphilis as a major public health concern in the 1950s and 1960s (and its reappearance as a major public health concern in the age of AIDS), the face of the syphilitic and the too small nose that marked it became a marginal marker of difference, much as the too small nose of the "leper" (Hansen's disease) or the person with scrofula did in the course of the nineteenth century.

Such images never truly vanish; they merely recede in importance. While the power of the pug nose or the too small nose or no nose should end with the discovery that syphilis could be cured in its initial stage by antibiotics such as penicillin and thus avoid the appearance of a stigma in the infected and their offspring, the power of the image of the face deformed by such a nose remains a part of the visual vocabulary of the unacceptable nose in Western culture.

There is an extraordinary episode of *The Twilight Zone*, by Rod Serling (1924–1975), seen on November 11, 1960, that plays on the association between such a deformed face and the world of aesthetic surgery. The episode begins with a shot of the bandaged face of Janey Tyler (played by Maxine Stuart as the bandaged patient and Donna Douglas as the "beautiful" patient), whose "hideously abnormal face has made her an outcast all of her life." This is her last chance to begin to "look normal."[7] We learn from monitors throughout the hospital that the Leader of the State wants "glorious conformity," and if she is not able to be transformed she will be banished to a village where others of her kind are forced to reside. We never see any of the faces of the staff or of the other patients in the hospital. When the bandages are removed we are shocked to see an extremely beautiful face. But the operation is declared a failure by the surgeon! We then see the hideous faces of the surgeons and the staff. As William Tuttle, the makeup man on the episode noted, "The idea was to make them look like pigs, with the big nostrils and the pig-like nose." Their "pig-like noses" are a clear evocation, whether conscious or not, of the pug nose that haunted the image of the syphilitic. Following the unsuccessful surgery, the patient is led off by an equally "handsome" man to the world of the "deformed." Strikingly, the title of the episode was "In the Eye of the Beholder."

Further, look at the cover of *Communion* (1989), a "memoir" of alien abduction by Whitley Strieber (1945–), and the 1989 film based on the novel, directed by Phillipe Mora and starring Christopher Walken.[8] The alien face that stares back at one is that of the Phantom. The description of the aliens captures virtually every image used by writers about "alien abductions": "Besides stocky beings, dressed in blue cover-all type suits, Strieber remembered others, one type being 'about five feet tall, very slender and delicate, with extremely prominent and mesmerizing black slanted eyes . . . and most vestigial mouth and nose.' Others had round eyes."[9] In another account, there were some with "wide faces, appearing either dark gray or dark blue, with glittering deep-set eyes, pug noses, and broad, somewhat human mouths."[10] This is the stuff of nightmares, of being entered and polluted by an alien force, whether syphilis or the inhabitant of the space ship. The terror is captured in the face of the "alien." One case study should suffice: "A psychiatrist told me about a patient of hers, 'a high-functioning woman professional,' who began to suffer anxiety attacks after seeing the face of the 'alien' on the cover of Whitley Strieber's book *Communion*. Under hypnosis and in 'spontaneous flashbacks' she had recalled multiple encounters with and gynecological exams by similar-appearing 'aliens.'"[11] The sexual import of the alien's face (Strieber himself claimed to have been anally raped by his captors) is a continuation of the sexual anxiety focused on the face of the syphilitic.

6. The Role of Aesthetics in Creating

the Psyche

What happens when everyone in a society is finally beautiful (and healthy)? When the final aesthetic surgery is developed that will make all visages and bodies "perfect"? Will everyone in that society be happy? In examining the discourses of the late nineteenth century on this question, we are confronted with the paradox of François Xavier Bichat (1771–1802), as paraphrased by Charles Darwin: "If every one were cast in the same mould, there would be no such thing as beauty. If all our women were to become as beautiful as the Venus de' Medici [de Milo], we should for a time be charmed; but we should soon wish for variety; and as soon as we had obtained variety, we should wish to see certain characters a little exaggerated beyond the then existing common standard."[1] The very search for the improvement of the body (and the concomitant "happiness" of the psyche) must lead to further discontent. Passing as a member of the "beautiful," and therefore, healthy class means diluting that class into the "normal." This is the negative aspect of the Enlightenment promise of transformation—when everyone is transformed, passing can have no value. Except, of course, for those who are racially passing. For Bichat, whose science supported the notion of a "blood consciousness," passing was impossible and would lead to disaster and further unhappiness.

And yet the contravening view was also present. Operate upon the body and make the psyche happy. Unhappiness, melancholy, sadness, anger—all of these negative feelings that can be corrected by aesthetic surgery—vanish when everyone is beautiful and identifiably healthy, when no one is seen as deviating from the norm. But beauty quickly becomes the desired norm. And yet the uniformity of beauty comes to destroy its own objective—the perfection of the soul.

The sense is that one vanishes into the beautiful, the good, the healthy—that this category defines (in)visibility. This may seem counterintuitive. Does not the aesthetic surgery patient desire to stand out as "beautiful" and does not this extraordinary ability provide the claim for happiness? Are you not happy when you are more beautiful? What the beautiful comes to mean is vital for our examination of the psychological underpinning of aesthetic surgery. When beauty (however defined) becomes the norm for the idealized person, beauty is associated with other forms of perfection, such as moral character and aesthetic creativity. In such a world beauty is not the exception in this idealized worldview, rather, the beautiful is the norm.

Karl Rosenkranz (1805-1879), Hegel's best-known student, justified his undertaking an aesthetics of the ugly by stating in his introduction that the study of the ugly is to the examination of beauty what the study of pathology is to illness.[2] For him the aesthetics of the body were also the aesthetics of medicine. The medical analogy—the exploration of the dead body as a means of understanding the living one is parallel to the study of the ugly body as a means of understanding the beautiful one—is central to his analysis, as the pathological came to be understood as the ugly. Illness, deformity, loss of function, aging, malproportion, infection, risk—all of these categories that define deviancy from the healthy norm in medical thought become one with the notion of the ugly. Deviancy is understood as making the individual unhappy.

In Rosenkranz's aesthetics of the ugly, the "ugly" is dependent on the essential nature of "beauty." "Beauty," like "goodness," for him, is an absolute category; "ugliness," like "evil," is a relative category. Likewise, illness is understood in the medical (and pathological) literature of the nineteenth century as dependent in its definition on the definition of the normal.[3] The healthy are the baseline for any definition of the acceptable human being, as if the changes of the body, labeled as illness or aging or disability, were foreign to the definition of the "real" human being. Only the healthy are happy.

Our present sense of a normative beauty or a standard of handsomeness is established for the modern period by the Enlightenment (as is its critique); this Enlightenment norm begins to see the beautiful as the baseline for the acceptable body (as it also sees the ugly as the definition of the unacceptable).[4] Such an elision of the "beautiful" with the "body" is clearly anti-Platonic, for Plato stressed that the vision of divine beauty was free from "any taint of human flesh" (*Symposium* 211e). Like Empedocles's "alien garb of flesh," the physical is separate and distinct from abstractions such as the good, the beautiful, and the healthy.[5] But the Platonic ideal of a beauty freed from the body was not the dominant concept in the beginning of our modern confrontation with the body. Even neo-Platonism as filtered through Pauline Christianity equated "matter," the material body, with evil, with the ugly, and with disease. The body came to define the representation of "beauty" and "ugliness" in the world. And the body also defined the line between the "happy" and the "unhappy," the "moral" and the "immoral." All was written on the body.

In the Enlightenment Immanuel Kant articulated the general premise that aesthetic judgment was not a rational but an affective judgment. It is the "feeling [of the internal sense] of the concept in the play of the mental powers as a thing only capable of being felt."[6] And yet this sense is conceived by each of us, according to Kant, as universal, and we "lay claim to the concurrence of everyone, whereas no private sensation would be decisive except for the observer alone" (73). We see the world of beauty (and health) as necessarily greater than we are, and yet these concepts are rooted in our own experience. When Kant imagines the power of the aesthetic as captured in the plastic arts, he stresses that it is an affective rather than an intellectual force. It demands that one imagine a shared and naive universality, for the plastic arts presents "concepts of things corporeally, as they might exist in nature" (186). Thus when aesthetic surgeons sought for models of the beautiful body during the nineteenth century, it was to the plastic arts that they turned. Kant divided "nature" into "physiology," i.e., the way that "nature made man," and "anthropology," i.e., "what man has made of himself." The latter became the space where aesthetic surgery could be imagined.

In addition, for Kant, in the aesthetic discussion in the first half of the *Critique of Judgment* (1790), the aesthetic is also a moral category because both the "beautiful" and the "good" please the self.[7] Thus aesthetic feelings provide "happiness," which is an emotional rather than a cognitive quality. Corporeality becomes the basis for the understanding of the beautiful and the ugly, for the healthy and the ill.

For Kant or Rosenkranz, the norms of the beautiful/ugly—like the norms of the healthy/ill—are not bound to any culture. Therefore, disease, too, forms a universal category of aesthetic evaluation. In his discussion, Rosenkranz focuses on the deformed as his category of the diseased. The deformed is that structure of human existence that deviates from the norm of the beautiful (i.e., functional) body. Given Rosenkranz's position at the midpoint of the nineteenth century, just as Bénédict Auguste Morel (1809-1873) was formulating the notion of "degeneration" and Dieffenbach was sundering reconstructive from aesthetic surgery, it should be of little surprise that the aesthetics of the ugly and the diseased become a type of aesthetic degeneration theory. The existence of an a priori notion of the beautiful allows a limited number of possibilities for the existence of the ugly, just as the existence of an a priori notion of the healthy presents a limited range of possibilities for the existence of the diseased.

The dichotomy between the beautiful and the ugly seems to be inherent in all of the cultural constructs of health and disease in the nineteenth and twentieth centuries. By the end of the nineteenth century individual beauty comes to have significance as a sign of the healthiness of the race. Here, to no one's surprise, the notion of the healthy and beautiful race evolved into the discourse of eugenics, another form of hygiene. Francis Galton (1822–1911), Charles Darwin's cousin and the founder of eugenics as a "science," early in his career mapped Britain creating a "beauty map," calculating the ratio of attractive to plain to ugly women.[8] Galton's intent was to provide a basis for the selection of better spouses for his male audience. It is only the "new" science, here eugenics, that can restore the beauty of the body politic. "Race," however, is only a placeholder for the idea of the "healthy" and "beautiful" collective that must be preserved. Aesthetic surgery arises out of this world. It is a world, to cite Michel Foucault, built upon the Enlightenment ideals of "disciplining the body and of regulating populations."[9] The ugly and the diseased must give way to the beautiful and the healthy.

In an afterward to the turn-of-the-century study of "social disease" by Jules Héricourt (1850–?), his British translator Bernard Miall provided the reader with the ultimate rationale for the control and exclusion of the sick from the body politic. It is not only the need to separate the healthy from the sick, but equally to isolate the beautiful from the ugly, the happy from the unhappy:

> We need a religion of beauty, of perfection. It would be a simple matter to teach children to worship perfection rather than hate it because it reveals their own imperfection. For we cannot teach what beauty is without making plain the hideousness of egoism. Beauty is the outward and visible sign of health—perfection—virtue. Pleasure is the perception of beauty, or some of its elements. What makes for the fullness and perfection of life, for beauty and happiness, is good; what makes for death, disease, imperfection, suffering, is bad. These things are capable of proof, and a child may understand them. Sin is ugly and painful. Perfection is beautiful and gives us joy. We have appealed to the Hebraic conscience for two thousand years in vain. Let us appeal to the love of life and beauty which is innate in all of us. A beauty-loving people could not desire to multiply a diseased or degenerate strain, or hate men and women because they were strong and comely and able. . . . The balance of the races is overset, and only the abandonment of voluntary sterility by the fit, and its adoption by the unfit— which is eugenics—can save us.[10]

Miall's view echoes an association of the healthy with the beautiful that acquired its most explicit statement at the close of the nineteenth century. It is a restatement of a commonplace from the ancients to the moderns.

Physical attractiveness, however culturally defined, came to be seen as a sign of virtue. Moral goodness, "calocagathia," came to be seen as inscribed on the body. Cicero had written that "it matters greatly to the soul by what sort of body it is placed; for there are many conditions of the body that sharpen the mind, and many that blunt it."[11] And Lavater, the Swiss physiognomist, recapitulated this at the close of the eighteenth century, noting that "the beauty and deformity of the countenance is in just and determinate proportion to the moral beauty and deformity of the man. The morally best, the most beautiful. The morally worst, the most deformed."[12] It is not only that the healthy becomes the beautiful, but the beautiful becomes the healthy; the diseased is not only the ugly, but the ugly the diseased.[13] Also, the ugly must be made to give way to the beautiful through the agency of scientific medicine such as aesthetic surgery. What is desired is a world peopled by the beautiful, and only an absolute norm of beauty is permitted. Such beauty permits the individual experiencing it to be happy.

Certainly the connection drawn by Johann Joachim Winckelmann (1717-1768) between the "beauty of the Greeks" and the "beauty of their art" made the ugly and the nonproductive into linked categories.[14] Yet Winckelmann was clear that it was *only* with the Greeks that one had a world in which the "beautiful people" dominated. His Germany as well as his Italy was filled with people who were simply ordinary—neither beautiful nor grotesque. Reconstituting the world of the Greeks meant re-creating a world of beautiful, happy people at one with their bodies and psyches. This is the fantasy that haunts the background of aesthetic surgery.

The antithesis to this new vocabulary of aesthetic perfection is, according to Miall, the old and faulty promise of conscience and religion, with its "Hebraic conscience." In starkly Nietzschean terms, Miall defines the brave new world of European (defined as British if you are in Britain; German if you are in Germany; French if you are in France) science against religion, here Christianity, the European legacy of the Jews. This move is not an accidental one. With the rise of materialism within medicine, the struggle comes to be between "theology" (ugly) and "science" (beauty), and Nietzsche reads this as an overcoming of the Jewish (read: ugly) aspect of the modern soul. The Jew is the very model of the ugly and the diseased. Nietzsche argued in *The Genealogy of Morals* (1887) that "it was the Jew who, with frightening consistency, dared to invert the aristocratic value equations good/noble/powerful/beautiful/happy/favored-of-the-god and maintain that only the poor, the powerless, are good; only the suffering, sick, and ugly, truly blessed."[15] The second half of this quotation is, of course, a summary of the Beatitudes, for

Christianity is merely Rabbinic Judaism in another guise. It is the weak, sickly, and ugly race that must give way to its antithesis, the strong, the healthy, the beautiful.

When translated into the discourse of the favored vs. the ill-favored races one major aspect of the aesthetics of health and illness surfaces. It is the association of the beautiful with the erotic; the ugly, with the unerotic. The unerotic or the unpleasurable must give way to the pleasure of the erotic. It is the attraction of the beautiful that will enable the race to maintain its beauty. These terms are unmistakably gendered. Thus in Héricourt's terms sterility is a social disease that makes the female, no matter how alluring on the surface, inherently ugly. Only the fecund are truly beautiful for they reproduce the race. In the discourse of health, the erotic comes to play a major role in defining the beautiful and the ugly.

Kant recognizes the categories of body form and healthy character as early as his essay on the sublime, when he writes concerning the nature of female beauty that the beautiful woman is defined by "a well proportioned figure, regular features, colors of eyes and face which contrast prettily, beauties pure and simple which are also pleasing in a bouquet and gain a cool approbation." This "beauty" is reflected in the character of the woman, for "the moral composition makes itself discernible in the mien or facial features, she whose features show qualities of beauty is *agreeable*, and if she is that to a high degree, *charming*."[16] Implied in Kant's argument is "youthfulness," which defines the erotic. If, as Kant argues, the female defines the beautiful, the link between beauty and health (defined as reproductive ability) is clear. Only the beautiful should be able to or would want to reproduce.

Such beauty must be universal: "I affirm that the sort of beauty we have called the pretty figure is judged by all men very much alike. . . . The Turks, the Arabs, the Persians are apparently of one mind in this taste, because they are very eager to beautify their races through such fine blood [of Circassian and Georgian maidens]" (89). The cultural significance of these views in late-nineteenth-century Europe is clear.[17] It is not only that these physical signs of difference are taken to have diagnostic value. That which is "ill-proportioned, irregular, non-contrastive" is not only ill, but will make the society as a whole ill. From the eighteenth century, those defined as "not German" in Germany, such as the Jews, are seen as having darker or yellowish skin color and often are labeled as having a body form that reveals their potential for illness.

By the nineteenth century male Jews are seen as feminized, belonging to an "inferior race."[18] The Jew, in his "absence of creative power, of spontaneity and of originality . . . displays in this respect something of a woman's nature. The Semites are said to be a feminine race, possessing to a high degree the gift of receptivity, always lacking in virility and procreative power" (247). The visualization of the difference of the male Jew is thus in terms of this image of the unproductive and the ill, specifically the image of the tubercular female, who is simultaneously "beautiful" (but dangerous) and "diseased." Here Rosenkranz's image comes full circle in categorizing the apparent rejection of the Jew as a figure of desire in post-Enlightenment Europe.

The Jew's "bodily infirmity" is marked by the Jew's "unmanly appearance." He is like but not identical to the tubercular woman, specifically the tubercular Jewish woman. The Jew's visage is like "those lean actresses, the *Rachels* and *Sarahs*, who spit blood, and seem to have but the spark of life left, and yet who, when they have stepped upon the stage, put forth indomitable strength and energy. Life, with them, has hidden springs" (150). It is the tubercular Jewish woman that the healthy male Jew looks like. It is Sarah Bernhardt (1844–1923) and Rachel Félix (1820–1858), the two best-known Jewish actresses on the nineteenth-century Parisian stage, both tubercular, who mark the essence of the normal physiognomy of the *male* Jew. Jewish women, for example, are rarely considered to be "agreeable" or "charming."

And yet why is it, Kant asks, that "many women" have a liking for "a healthy but pale color," which should, he implies, be a sign of pathology? "This generally accompanies a disposition of more inward feeling and delicate sensation, which belongs to the quality of the sublime; whereas the rosy and blooming complexion proclaims less of the first, but more of the joyful and merry disposition—but it is more suitable to vanity to move and to arrest, than to charm and to attract" (88). Again it is character that is mirrored in the face, but it is not the face of the pathological, only that which evokes or affirms the possibility of that which is greater than the self, the sublime. The aesthetic qualities often ascribed to the ill ("delicacy") come to signal a type of character that is merely a variation on the beautiful, rather than its antithesis. This problem of distinguishing between the truly sick and the truly healthy, the truly beautiful and the truly ugly, is never resolved by the philosophers of the age.

In the general medical literature on degeneracy, the signs of beauty and ugliness are usually gendered in quite a different manner. "Plumpness," as I have shown elsewhere, has a double-edged meaning at the turn of the century: it is a sign of stability but also, potentially, a sign of satiety and sexuality.[19] "Normal" women, to use the distinction made by Cesare Lombroso (1835–1909), can be plump and are therefore healthy; "criminal women, such as prostitutes" are plump, a sign of their "natural" tendency to their craft. It is important to note that the contexts for the reading of the physiognomy are absolutely clear—one knows whether the sign of plumpness means danger or succor. Chronologically, however, and here the notion of degeneracy again rears its head, it is impossible to tell. We know, says Lombroso's Russian colleague Pauline Tarnowsky, that even the most beautiful prostitute will eventually reveal her degenerate physiognomy, for what is within will—indeed, must—out.

Certainly this image of beauty as the mask of a dangerous, that is, infectious or contagious, illness affects the representation of the body of the tubercular in the nineteenth and twentieth centuries. So there was a need to unmask the hidden pathology under the skin. Can surgery so alter the body that it will not become ill and thus remain happy? If not, can we at least identify visually those bodies that have a potential for illness? Questions of "constitution" and "body type" attempt to reveal the hidden illness well before the illness manifests itself.

There is no clearer pattern for the relationship between an idealized body type and an "ugly," that is, potentially ill, body type than in the ancient question of whether people with a specific body type are predisposed to acquiring tuberculosis. The *habitus phthisicus* was the clearest sign for an "inherited diathesis," a predisposition to tuberculosis, as early as the times of Hippocrates and Galen. Indeed, in the eighteenth century, Friedrich Hoffmann (1660–1742) believed that "tall people with long necks" were prone to tuberculosis.[20] This tradition of the ugly as a sign of disease is stressed in the classic history of constitutional theory that opened the standard fin de siècle periodical on the topic.[21] The ugly may not be immediately ill, but their deformed bodies predispose them to illness. They hide within them the roots of the destruction of the collective, because if they reproduce, their body type will predispose their offspring to illness. No exercise, no surgery, no cosmetics will change this.

And yet the desire was to find a way out of the dilemma, to provide for the pursuit of happiness promised by the Enlightenment—and aesthetic surgery was the result of this pursuit. All of the treatments of the psyche through the alteration of the body in the course of the nineteenth and early twentieth centuries relied on the presupposition of an aesthetics of the body in which there was an absolute relationship to the psyche. What manifested itself in the mind was written upon the body; what appeared on the body shaped the mind. These are some of the complexities of imagining a psychology of aesthetic surgery.

Part Two

Too Many Psyches

1. John Orlando Roe's Pragmatic
Psychology

When the first aesthetic surgeons began to practice what we today recognize as the antecedents to the contemporary procedures of aesthetic surgery, they saw themselves as the natural continuation of the faciomaxillary and plastic surgeons who grafted and reconstructed faces and bodies during the nineteenth century. These surgeons, such as Dieffenbach, the German facial surgeon, had to overcome the stigma of working with patients, such as the Phantom of the Opéra, recognizably suffering from stigmatizing diseases such as syphilis.[1] These surgeons' procedures, such as the use of grafts to replace missing noses, were seen as radical because they attempted to alter signs that were unmistakably supposed to mark the immoral, unclean, and polluted. They were often condemned by the more traditional medical establishment, who were anxious not to be associated with quacks of any stripe. Slowly, with the establishment of the field of "plastic surgery" (a term introduced during the 1830s) as a "serious" specialty within surgery, Dieffenbach and his contemporaries came to define the accepted boundaries of aesthetic surgery. By the 1880s it was clear that surgical procedures could be performed on bodies that by Dieffenbach's definition were functionally "healthy." Surgical alterations of the face were done at the behest of the patients, often with clear directions as to the type of alterations they desired.

To defend themselves against the charge of violating the Hippocratic Oath by operating on healthy patients, surgeons began to understand their medical practice as a form of somatopsychological therapy. They were altering the body to change the psyche. In 1887 John Orlando Roe (1849–1915) in Rochester, New York, developed a procedure to alter the shape of the "pug nose."[2] Roe did not claim only to cure the "pug nose"; he claimed also to be curing his patient's unhappiness. His comprehension of the relationship between mind and body was clear: "We are able to relieve patients of a condition which would remain a lifelong mark of disfigurement, constantly observed, forming a never ceasing source of embarrassment and mental distress to themselves, amounting, in many cases, to a positive torture, as well as often causing them to be objects of greater or lesser aversion to others. . . . The effect upon the mind of such physical defects is readily seen reflected in the face, which invariably conforms to the mental attitude, and leads after a time to a permanent distortion of the countenance."[3] Thus a double physiognomy was present in such patients. They had a deformity (according to their own account), and this deformity caused them psychological discomfort. In turn this discomfort altered their physiognomy so that they looked not only deformed but also unhappy. The surgeon, in curing the deformity, makes the patient happy, which in turn alters the physiognomy. The model of the patient's psyche is quite simple: the deformity affects the conscious mind through the patient's reception in society. The operation alters the perception of the body in others and thus alters the patient's consciousness. Everything takes place in the conscious mind. The surgeon's model is a very simple psychological loop.

One central problem was the seeming nonmedical notion of the patient's autonomy. For it is the patient who initiates and defines treatment. In his 1892 paper on "sunken noses," Robert F. Weir (1838–1894) presented a case of "monomania" focusing on the nose.[4] The nose that Weir repaired, however, was not a flattened, pug nose, but rather a nose that was "unduly large." The male patient came to Weir in 1887 "perturbed in mind concerning the unsightliness of his nose." This was not merely a "cosmetic annoyance"; rather, "his physicians and relatives [saw it as] essential to the preservation of the balance of his mind." The shape of the nose was altered by the removal of a section of the septum intranasally. "The patient's mental relief was correspondingly great for a time." A few months after the correction, the patient returned wanting the nose to be reshaped. This was done with an incision that altered the form of the base of the nose. A year later the patient again returned requesting another operation. Weir initially refused because he "considered it a first-class nose as it was," but he was again per-suaded by his patient's family (141–42). A further intranasal opera-tion followed. Weir is perplexed that the surgeon's intervention, which created a "normal" nose, was not sufficient for the patient. He seems to have fulfilled the request of the family and the patient by having "cured" his psyche, and yet the now "normal" nose (as judged by the surgeon based on the limitations of his techniques) still made the patient unhappy. Can surgery truly cure unhappi-ness, or does it lead to ever greater demands for its impossible cure?

An answer of sorts was supplied by Jacques Joseph (1865–1934), a highly acculturated young German Jewish surgeon practicing in fin de siècle Berlin. In January 1898, a twenty-eight-year-old man came to him with the complaint that "his nose was the source of considerable annoyance. Wherever he went, everybody stared at him; often, he was the target of remarks or ridiculing gestures. On account of this he became melancholic, withdrew almost com-pletely from social life, and had the earnest desire to be relieved of this deformity."[5] Joseph altered the shape of his patient's nose. On May 11, 1898, he reported on this operation before the Berlin Medical Society. In that report Joseph provided a detailed "scien-tific" rationale for performing a medical procedure on what was an otherwise completely healthy individual: "The psychological effect of the operation is of utmost importance. The depressed attitude of the patient subsided completely. He is happy to move around unnoticed. His happiness in life has increased, his wife was glad to report; the patient who formerly avoided social contact now wishes to attend and give parties. In other words, he is happy over the results."[6] The anomaly of the "unhappy" patient, which Joseph deals with later in his career, is explained as a too heightened sen-sitivity to beauty.

Joseph comments on Weir's patient noting that he "felt very un-happy on account of his somewhat protruding nose" (167). The sub-sequent corrections that Weir makes are seen as necessary because of the less successful nature of the surgeon and his procedure, not as a reflex of the patient's insatiable demand for perfection: "Robert Weir's case and mine are similar. . . . On the other hand, they differ considerably in the surgical method, and especially in the success, which in my case was achieved in a single operation, without any secondary corrections" (167). The "normal" patient's expectations match the surgeon's ability and thus both are happy with the results.

In 1904 Joseph commented on the psychology of his male patients whom he successfully cured of their psychological difficulties: "The patients were embarrassed and self-conscious in their dealings with their fellow men, often shy and unsociable, and had the urgent desire to become free and unconstrained. Several complained of sensitive drawbacks in the exercise of their profession. As executives they could hardly enforce their authority; in their business connections (as salesmen, for example), they often suffered material losses. . . . The operative nasal reduction—this is my firm conviction—will also in the future restore the joy of living to many a wretched creature and, if his deformity has been hindering him in his career, it will allow him the full exercise of his aptitudes."[7] According to Joseph the patient "is happy to move around unnoticed." Surgery restores or creates "happiness" and is therefore successful. Social roles determine happiness. Entering into the world as an (in)visible member of the "normal" society gave men the social status they need to be "real men." This move creates happiness and cures the psyche. Aesthetic surgery has taken its place among the specialties competing to cure the psyche at the turn of the century.

Joseph's understanding of the relationship between mind and body, that the correction of the body heals the psyche, is keyed to an understanding of his patients as inherently "healthy." Their visibility as a member of one cohort makes them ill; in a "normal," (in)visible state as a member of another cohort, they would be quite happy and therefore completely healthy. This is analogous to other discussions among the aesthetic surgeons of the late nineteenth century. It is clearest where the patient was understood by the physician to be psychopathic—where the alteration of the nose did not heal the psyche.

The demand for repeated surgery ("polysurgery") was to become a sign of psychopathology, as we shall see later in this section.[8] Such patients were never satisfied because they could never feel themselves as members of the "other" cohort. Such patients were used to draw the boundary between the professional domains of the aesthetic surgeon and that of the psychiatrist. Weir is one of the first surgeons to see repetition as a sign of the patient's failure of insight in having the "good enough nose." Yet the problem is much more complex than merely resolving the border disputes between medical subspecialties. What Joseph had learned with his insight about the meaning of the patient's (not the surgeon's) scars, is that anything that is perceived as making the patient identifiable as having been a member of another cohort vitiates the psychological impact of the surgery. Scarring, the experimental nature of the early procedures, even the change of surgical styles over time, cause the members of the "normal" cohort to comment on those who desire to pass. And this nullifies the attempt. Weir's patient signaled the ever increasing threshold for (in)visibility demanded by the aesthetic surgical patient.

Here we can evoke Jean-Jacques Rousseau (1712–1778), who commented in his novel of education, *Emile* (1762), that "the way in which the Author of our being has shaped our heads does not suit us; we must have them modeled from without by midwives and from within by philosophers."[9] For Joseph articulated the basic premise of modern aesthetic surgery, that the correction of perceived physical anomalies was a means of repairing not the body but the psyche. He did this at exactly the same moment in modern history that Sigmund Freud had begun to understand the basis for his own approach for curing the hysterical body, with all of its physical signs and symptoms, through the treatment of the psyche. Aesthetic surgery comes to be understood as "somatopsychic therapy" in which "it is exclusively the altered or defective form of the pathologically and anatomically normal organ that causes psychic conflicts."[10] We see at the close of the nineteenth century a "modeling from within" by physicians rather than philosophers. What if, however, the source of the dis-ease with one's body comes as much from an internalization of the society's image of oneself as from any private cause? What if the anti-Semitic representation of the Jewish nose—so widely present in the literature of the fin de siècle —itself shaped the Jew's response to the Jew's own nose? It is in this context that the damaged psyche of the Jew was to be repaired.

We must pause at this point and ask: What is it that makes these "pug-nosed" and "large-nosed" individuals unhappy? Dieffenbach notes that people without noses were believed to be suffering from syphilis, no matter what the actual etiology of their deformity. A decade or so after Dieffenbach, the meaning of the "pug nose" in Rochester, New York, and the meaning of the "large nose" in Berlin and New York had changed radically. Here the question of stigma was tied to the representation of ethnic difference. The "pug nose" was the Irish nose, well represented in the caricatures of the age; the "large nose," as we shall discuss in detail below, was the visual icon of the Jew. No longer was "disease" the thing that people wanted to hide (though it is clear that the stigma of the syphilitic "facies" continues well into the twentieth century), but rather their ethnic identity. The origins of modern procedures in the closing decades of the nineteenth century, from the modern rhinoplasty to abdominal reduction, were all nuanced by the anxiety about the racial body and the racial character.

The promise of Enlightenment autonomy that one could change one's identity by altering the body was one that the aesthetic surgeons attempted to fulfill. Once the form of the nose becomes a key to seeing character, the nose may place an individual in a cohort where he or she does not want to belong. Individuals with a pug nose may "look Irish" even though they are not. The ability to pass was thus coupled with the anxiety of being perceived as different.

2. Enrico Morselli's Dysmorphophobia

Curing the psyche at the end of the nineteenth century was a contested arena. The neurologists (and later psychoanalysts), such as Sigmund Freud, laid claim to their ability to cure their idea of the psyche by seeing it as a reflex of the nervous system. The psychiatrists (or alienists) such as Richard von Krafft-Ebing (1840–1902) laid claim to their ability to cure their understanding of the psyche out of their reasonably recent responsibility for running asylums and for defining the phenomenon of psychopathology in the courts. Finally the aesthetic surgeons claimed that they could cure their image of the psyche by operating on the body. The explicit answer of the psychoanalysts to the cure of the psyche came in the first decade of the twentieth century as aesthetic surgery was becoming popular. But the response of late-nineteenth-century clinical psychiatry evolved exactly as the first procedures called aesthetic surgery in the closing decades of the nineteenth century were being developed.[1]

The answer of the clinical psychiatrists was formulated by a later correspondent of Freud, Enrico Morselli (1852–1929). Morselli coined the diagnostic category of "dysmorphophobia" in 1891, although he made reference to an earlier paper from 1886 in which he began to discuss such concepts.[2] The key to the acceptance of Morselli's paper was that it appeared to be presented within the phenomenological discourse of scientific psychiatry that had begun to dominate European psychiatry through the work of German psychiatrists. The ideology was that diagnostic categories, like biological ones, were "natural," merely outlining the set of fixations that characterized this syndrome. It was as if Morselli had discovered a natural entity and was "objectively" describing it. Yet when his act of description is examined, it is clear that there is a similar physiognomic model to that used empirically by the aesthetic surgeons, such as Roe, Weir, and Joseph, in the 1880s and 1890s. These surgeons, in the United States and in Germany, were beginning to think about altering the racial body to relieve unhappiness. But does the alteration of the body actually change one's "racial" psyche? For it is not only the body, but also the character that theories of race claimed were fixed.[3] Surgeons and patients were all working with a specific notion of the relationship between the psyche and the body.

In his paper, Morselli stressed the fixed physiognomy of the patient as the focus of the patient's unhappiness. He described the patients' fixation on specific qualities of that body: the low and mashed forehead, the absurd nose, and the bandy legs (111). These qualities provided a physiognomic vocabulary for both the clinical psychiatrists and their patients. The racial physiognomy in this description is self-evident from the cultural images of the time. Morselli's image of the dysmorphic face is that of the African!

For specific readings of the meaning of this physiognomy we can turn to Morselli's teacher at the Instituto de Studi Superiori in Florence in the 1870s, the late-nineteenth-century Italian physician and theorist Paolo Mantegazza (1831–1910). In his widely cited fin de siècle account of physiognomy, he stressed: "We, belonging to the higher races, regard as ugly all noses which approach that of the ape, snub, flattened, or very small noses, with nostrils failing in parallelism, and the section of which represents the figure eight. In this respect we even sacrifice the laws of geometry to our atavistic prejudices; we should consider a woman beautiful who had an excessively large nose, rather than pardon a snub one. In Italy we call a large nose aristocratic (especially if it is aquiline), perhaps because the long-nosed conquerors, Greek or Latin, subjugated the autocthonous small-nosed population."[4] Here it is the long nose of the Italian that is contrasted with the "ape-like" nose that marked the "lower species." And this is the "ridiculous" nose that accompanies the low forehead and bandy legs that compose the physical stereotype of the African in late-nineteenth-century thought. Morselli (and his patients) cannot imagine a more horrific image than seeing oneself as potentially black. One might add that Morselli not only studied physiognomy under Mantegazza but also studied phrenology under the tutelage of the anthropologist Paolo Gaddi (?–1872). His concept of the relationship of mind to body and of the reading of the fixed physiognomy of the body was clearly indebted to both of these teachers. Yet it was cast in the phenomenological language of the new clinical psychiatry of the late nineteenth century.

Morselli's sources for his category of dysmorphophobia are all taken from German clinical literature of the time. His authorities are Emil Kraepelin (1856–1926) and Krafft-Ebing, both of whom he cites. He creates this nosological category as part of a major shift in the meaning of obsessive neurosis. The older, materialistic view, such as that held by Freud's teacher Theodor Meynert (1833–1892) (in a key essay published in 1888), saw it as an organic brain disturbance that defied any and all treatment.[5] The "newer" view in the 1890s, espoused by neurologists such as Freud as well as clinical psychiatrists such as Theodor Ziehen (1862–1950), made a differential diagnosis between obsessive neurosis and psychosis. They saw obsessive neurosis as a separate category of neurotic psychopathologies that could be "treated." Dysmorphophobia is shaped by Morselli's readings of this "new" reading of obsessive neurosis. Like the aesthetic surgeons who claimed to be able to cure the unhappy psyche, sufferers from dysmorphophobia could be cured using the classical treatments of the late-nineteenth-century alienist.

The shift from Meynert's idea of obsessive neurosis as an "untreatable" brain disorder to the image of it as a treatable neurosis has a hidden reading. The racial underpinning of this category is keyed to the understanding, implicit in nineteenth-century clinical psychiatry, that there is a "neurotic" group that by its "inbreeding" is least able to cope with the "modern." This group suffers most from all forms of mental illness, especially the anxiety about the body. The racial touchstone for the neurotic in both (the politically conservative) Kraepelin and (the politically liberal) Krafft-Ebing is not the African but the Jew. For both, the Jew is the representative of disease, inherently corrupt and only on the surface seemingly "healthy." They are the ones essentially obsessed by the nature of their bodies.

Krafft-Ebing's standard textbook of psychiatry, one of Morselli's sources, simply stated the "fact" that "Jews are especially prone to nervousness."[6] Kraepelin, the dean of fin de siècle German psychiatrists and professor of psychiatry at Munich, spoke with authority about the "domestication" of the Jews, their isolation from nature and their exposure to the stresses of modern life.[7] In his standard textbook, the Bible of German phenomenological psychiatry, he observes that there is a racial predisposition to mental illness among Jews in Germany and blacks in North America (1: 153–54). Race is a major qualifier in nineteenth-century clinical psychiatry. It also figures heavily in the representation of the accounts of cases of dysmorphophobia. Thus the claim is that no matter how mad the Jews are and no matter how obsessed they are with their bodies, clinical psychiatry offers the potential for a cure. When Kraepelin included dysmorphophobia as one of the compulsive neuroses, he stressed (following Morselli) the anxiety about having something "obvious or comical" about one's body such as (and this is his list in his order) "an unusually formed nose, knock-knees, a disgusting odor."[8] All of these are understood as defining aspects of the Jewish body at the fin de siècle.

The visualization of the imaginary Jew needed to be made concrete. The French turn-of-the-century anti-Semitic pamphleteer "Dr. Celticus" presents an anatomy of the Jew in which the "hooked nose" represents the "true Jew." "Nostrility" here becomes the first visual representation of the "primitiveness of the Semitic race."[9] How could one not be ashamed of such a face and such a body, whether one was a Jew or not, for it was a body that revealed the primitive nature of the character and psyche within. In Paris at the same moment, the anti-Semitic critic of psychoanalysis Pierre Janet (1859–1947) labeled this sense of discomfort with the body an "obsession with the shame of the body, the face, and the genitalia."[10] He saw it as a common experience of being shamed by the "ugly and ridiculous" nature of one's body. Janet moves his argument through a series of case studies. He begins with the obsession with gait in a male and moves to the qualities of the face, specifically the fantasies about the syphilitic face, in a female patient (359). Gait, too, is a sign of syphilitic infection. He concludes by examining sexual inversion as a form of obsessive neurosis focusing on the genitalia (365). Janet's cases center about symptoms that have been given meaning because of their function as "signs" of specific categories of pathology in the late nineteenth century. Whether they are "obsessive" because of that or for other reasons can never be determined. Janet's categories are never independent of such cultural qualities. For example, in the same work, he reiterates the predisposition of the Jews to various forms of mental illness (34) and stresses their inheritance of this predisposition (86).

This was the very moment when aesthetic surgery had begun to be understood as surgery on the psyche. Morselli's concept quickly came to be widely used in Europe, as the category of a mental illness in which there was a preoccupation with some imagined defect in appearance in a "normal"-appearing person or the exaggeration of a slight physical anomaly ("normal"-appearing to the psychiatrist, of course). The term is introduced into English with the publication of Eugenio Tanzi's (1856–?) Italian textbook in 1910, just at the very beginning of the rapid spread of aesthetic surgery in the United States.[11]

One might add that Enrico Morselli came to be well known for his anti-Semitic attitudes.[12] In 1926 he wrote a two-volume study that argued that psychoanalysis was a Jewish discovery because of the predisposition of the Jews to finding theoretical solutions for material problems. Freud detested Morselli's *La psicanalisi: Studii ed appunti critici*, noting in a letter to Edoardo Weiss that its "only value is its undoubted proof that he is a donkey. It contains numerous large and small mistakes. . . . Furthermore, it is covered by a layer of false courtesy, as used to be characteristic for the *Katzelmacher* [pejorative term for Italian] in old Austria." Freud's letter, phrased in equally obsequious terms, should be read in this context. Weiss, on Freud's behest, savaged the book both in German and in Italian reviews.[13] It is important to note the extraordinary ambivalence in Freud's response to Morselli and in his damning note on Morselli to Weiss.

Freud also ironically answered Morselli by claiming that Morselli's psychiatry was shaped by the major Jewish thinker of nineteenth-century Italian science, Cesare Lombroso. In 1926 Freud wrote to Morselli that while he does not know whether his thesis that "psychoanalysis as a direct product of the Jewish mind is correct, I would however not be ashamed if it were. Although long alienated from the religion of my ancestors, I have a feeling of solidarity with my people [*Volk*] and think with pleasure of that fact that you are a student of a man of my race [*Stammesgenossen*], the great Lombroso."[14] In other words, you are just about as Jewish as I am in the nature of your science! The connection between the Lombrosian theories of degeneration and Morselli's psychiatry are striking, but one must add that Lombroso did not believe that the alteration of the stigmata of the degenerate's body would, in any way, change the degenerate's character. Morselli's idea of a category for the diagnosis and cure of the neurotic's fixation on the body is a break with degeneracy theory. The origin of this seems to be in response to the claims of aesthetic surgery. Aesthetic surgeons believed they could operate upon the body and remove the stigmata of degeneration, such as the shape of the nose or the form of the ear. They claimed that such changes would actually alter the psyche of the individual.

It is clear that the clinical psychiatrists in the drive for a "pure phenomenology" of psychopathology avoided making "overt" readings of the symptoms they described. But their covert reading of what makes a "ridiculous" body had a contemporary, psychoanalytic reading in the work of one of the most orthodox of Freud's followers, Wilhelm Stekel (1868–1940). In his *Compulsion and Doubt* (1927) Stekel provided a reading of dysmorphophobia that places it in its contemporary context. (We will see in the course of this history of the psychologies in aesthetic surgery how the physician's definition of the question of the patient's motivation is central to the perceived success or failure of treatment.) He considered dysmorphophobia as part of those "compulsive ideas which concern the body," but which very specifically focus on a single aspect of the body.[15] While he begins with a general litany of body parts, "the nose, the bald head, the ear or (in women) the bosom" (1: 131), he very quickly selects two body parts that for him are determinant of this neurosis: the nose (in men) and the breasts (in women). He notes that no man ever obsesses about having a "beautiful" nose, only about the idea that "'I have a nose which is 'too big,' or 'too ugly,' or 'too Jewish-looking,' or 'asymmetrical.'" These three qualities (big, ugly, asymmetrical) defined the racial (Jewish) nose. Such patients define everything in "terms of 'nose currency,' he thinks in 'nose currency,' . . . he sees only noses which he continuously compares with his own." Following the model we outlined earlier, the materialism of the Jew, defined by his nose, reduces the entire universe to "currency." Stekel postulates an association of the nose with the penis (following Freud's [and Fliess's] model as we shall discuss below): "This disorder occurs more frequently in men than in women, a fact which corresponds to the phallic nature of the nose. (*Ex naso viris hastam.*)" The quotation from Ovid, that the size of the penis is related to the size of the nose, is ironic. For the nose reveals the "castrated" (i.e., circumcised) nature of the man with the long nose, not his supposed potency. Here we see the reversal of the world of the positive "too big nose," described by Mantegazza, into a world where the "too large" nose is a "real" or "supposed" sign of the Jew. If your nose is large, you are imagined to be castrated/circumcised, whether you are a Jew or not.

For the woman the equivalent is an obsessive focus on her breasts. Stekel presents here a case study of a "girl, aged twenty-six, [who] suffers from the obsession that her breasts are overly large and that they are pendulous. She wants to have an operation done but the surgeons refused. . . . She only wished to speak of her breasts and to convince me she was justified in asking for an operation." The gendered parallel to the (male's) Jewish nose, read in terms of his circumcised penis, is the (racialized) pendulous breasts of the woman. The aesthetic surgeons accept the idea of the racial breast as a given. Jacques Joseph described the "anthropology" of the breast as basic to any discussion of aesthetic surgery of the breast: "Certain racial differences exist with regard to the shape and growth pattern of the breast. Whereas among Caucasians the hemispherical breast shape is the most common, the pointed breast shape seems to predominate among black women."[16] In this world, large, pendulous breasts are as much a mark of the primitive within the body as is the circumcised penis.

All of Stekel's views provide a psychological definition of obsessive neurosis in terms of the culture of the day. He departs from a category of clinical psychiatry and adds a level of meaning to the symptoms that the phenomenological psychiatrists seemed simply to list. By the 1920s the clinical psychiatrists and the surgeons had defined the field—both see the obsession with the body as "treatable" but each provides different models for treatment. Following Stekel, in 1930, the clinical psychiatrist Walter Jahrreis focused on the notion of a beauty hypochondria that focuses on "one aspect of the bodily experience, which is experienced as deformed, repulsive, unacceptable or ridiculous."[17] He tried to strip this category of the overt meaning added by psychoanalysis, but it was retained in all its nuances.

After the Shoah the overt and covert racial references in this diagnostic category appear to vanish, and the term comes to have "classical overtones." The German psychiatrist Hermann Stutte (1909–) (in 1957) coined the Thersites-Complex, named after the ugliest man in the Greek army at Troy. For him the syndrome was characterized by a compulsive sense of being seen as ugly because of a specific quality of the body.[18] Stutte chose the repulsive figure of Theristes, with his game foot, bandy legs, and repulsive expression, to characterize the syndrome. It is not coincidental that Thersites is also one of the most vicious figures in the *Iliad*. He defines the boundary between the ignoble and the noble, the ugly and the handsome. Most important, he is a figure who seems not at all aware of his ugliness. Homer's implied comparison is with the moral and handsome Achilles, whose physiognomy he carefully never depicts. This translates the dichotomy of racial beauty into a cultural, neoclassical vocabulary, one that was quite comfortable for German academics from Freud to the present.

In 1962 another seemingly phenomenological presentation of the syndrome was made by Heinz Dietrich who defined it as the anxiety of creating anger through one's aesthetic presence.[19] The views of the Hungarian Jewish physician Alfred Berndorfer, which were formulated at much the same time, stated that the Jews suffered because of the anxiety of being seen by those who threatened them. This "feeling was projected upon their faces, and the psychic problem aggravated their facial expressions."[20] This view absolutely parallels the construction of the psyche as described in the 1880s by John Orlando Roe. Such an anxiety would be read by the perpetrators after the Shoah as the Jew's fear of offending through their physical presence. The blame is always laid at the nose of the victim.

All of these psychic aberrations were understood as nondelusional, and therefore different in kind from the somatic delusions associated with a wide range of psychopathologies ranging from Korsekoff's Syndrome to schizophrenia.[21] These approaches were all related to a psychology of the "ugliness" of the body that believed that no surgical intervention could alter the individual's obsession with the body. Only the therapies provided by the clinical psychiatrist would be effective.

Dysmorphophobia is but one of the numerous fashionable clinical labels for the obsession of patients with their bodies that were employed in the 1920s. Such patients seemed just as well to fit into the category of the "neurasthenic." An aesthetic surgeon commented in 1929, "To say that these people are neurasthenics means nothing, for psychologists teach 'that most patients, in addition to their troubles of a more technical type are somewhat neurasthenic.'"[22] From the standpoint of clinical psychiatry, surgery could not cure these forms of "inferiority complex," which we shall discuss in more detail below; indeed, it was claimed that it would exacerbate it.

The aesthetic surgeons of the beginning of this century both knew and had to respond to the claims that the clinical psychiatrist made that their patients should really be psychiatric patients. The most famous aesthetic surgeon of his day, Jacques Joseph rated his patients on a psychological scale.[23] He began with the "hypo-aesthetic" (who are unfazed even by gross deformities), to the "ortho-aesthetics" (normals who can "objectively" evaluate their deformities) to the "hyper-aesthetic" (who are "extremely unhappy," "having a strongly-developed sense of beauty such as painters, sculptors . . . and others of an artistic nature"). Joseph further labels such highly obsessive patients as "para-aesthetic" (36). For him their "pathologic aesthetic sensibility" focused on "imagined deformities." They have "normal or even beautiful features" that do not need change. They are not psychopathological. Indeed, one might define them as the most normal in their heightened aesthetic sensibilities.

Yet, as in Weir's patients, the heightened desire for a "perfect body" may hold its own psychological cure. "Sometimes," he writes, "an insignificant alteration of the shape of the nose, almost a sham operation in retrospect, can have a beneficial psychological effect. I performed surgery in such a case in which the operation was recommended by an eminent psychiatrist" (37). Such marginal interventions, as those proposed by Joseph, are clearly psychotherapy through surgical intervention and are so labeled. They provide a surgical psychotherapy for dysmorphophobia, which the phenomenological psychiatry of the nineteenth and early twentieth centuries claimed for itself.

One possible analogy to this view of the relationship between a "placebo" operation and the reconstitution of mental health can be found in dermatological cosmetology. This is one of the new, turn-of-the-century fields of medicine that shaped modern aesthetic surgery. In 1892 one of the pioneers in the field, Edmund Saalfeld (1862–1930), saw his work as an adjunct to that of clinical psychiatry. He wrote concerning women's preoccupation with their hair: "In many ladies who are constitutionally neurotic dwelling on abnormalities of the hair becomes a fixed idea; in men this very seldom happens. . . . You can meet these exaggerated complaints successfully only by psychical treatment in addition to medicinal. . . . These pitiable individuals believe that even when this abnormal growth of hair is relatively slight, they attract general attention in the street, and that everybody is laughing at them; they feel themselves socially impossible. In order to restore the peace of mind to these people there is only one remedy, and that is the removal of the hypertrichosis."[24] The category of "obsessive neurosis" (fixed ideas) becomes one that can be treated by somatic as well as psychological interventions—if not by both simultaneously.

This view continues. Bernard H. Shulman in 1980 asks, "Is the patient mentally ill? If so, should the surgery be done anyway? With what precautions?"[25] The search for a clinical model to determine how one can negotiate between the demands of the surgeon and the psychiatrist lead to a number of controlled studies of just this question. In 1988 three Japanese aesthetic surgeons at the Fukuoka University took 25 randomly selected patients who desired aesthetic surgery and gave them a battery of psychological tests.[26] They determined that nineteen of these patients were "psychiatrically abnormal." Five presented with dysmorphophobia, five with personality disorders, one with schizophrenia, one was retarded, seven were neurotic, including obsessive-compulsive patients. In other words by randomly selecting 25 out of a pool of

5,826 patients who came into their clinic they diagnosed 76 percent of the patients as evidencing psychopathologies. They rejected thirteen cases for surgery including three dysmorphophobics, one with personality disorder, the schizophrenic, the retarded person, three who were diagnosed as neurotic, and four "normals." The eight psychiatrically abnormal patients who underwent surgery were generally "satisfied" with the result; of those not operated on, eleven showed an improvement of their symptoms through psychotherapy and agreed to forego surgery. The line here between "surgery" and "psychotherapy" was absolute. The implication was that one could have equal, if not improved, results in making potential surgical patients "happy" through psychiatric intervention. Yet all of these discussions provided few clues to alternative therapeutic models for making patients happy.

One might add that following Joseph there have been constant attempts to reconceptualize the psychological classifications of patients for aesthetic surgery. Most of these make some type of primary differential between rational and nonrational choice. Thus Clarkson and Stafford-Clark in 1959 distinguished between "psychotic (or insane)" and "non-psychotic (or sane)" responses to deformity.[27] For them, speaking at an international conference of "plastic" surgery, the example of the dysmorphophobic patient is one who "may come to the plastic surgeon, asking for a change in shape or size of their nose, and may then provide some of the most unhappy complications from the psychiatric point of view. Indeed subsequent attempts to kill themselves, or more rarely even the plastic surgeon, are not unknown" (493). However, their case example is of a "woman with a large nose" who also had a delusion that "the proportions of this organ suggested to all who saw her that she had an equally large penis and was in fact a man masquerading as a woman" (494). Following Joseph's model, she was given a reduction rhinoplasty, and while her delusions returned after a year, they had changed in form and focus. Here surgery was seen as an appropriate intervention for an "insane" fixation with the body. Mixed signals occur when the clinical psychiatrists meet the aesthetic surgeons. Even dysmorphophobia is thus not necessarily an indicator to the surgeon not to operate—even if you may put your own life at risk!

The "neurosis"/"psychosis" boundary that was followed in the

Stafford-Clark and Clarkson paper was still dominant in American psychiatry with the first *Diagnostic and Statistical Manual of Mental Disorders* (DSM) of the American Psychiatric Association (1952).[28] Thus the psychotics were those who had delusions about a "real" deformity and those suffering from dysmorphophobia, delusions about their "normal" anatomy. The neurotic responses ranged from the mentally healthy to the unstable to the immature and those with grave neuroses. The assumption here, and in much of this literature, was counter to Joseph's—that the more severe the mental illness (with dysmorphophobia marking that boundary), the less advisable was aesthetic surgery.

By 1980, with the introduction of the concept of "body dysmorphic disorder" into the *Diagnostic and Statistical Manual of Mental Disorders*, the turn to a psychiatric rather than an aesthetic surgical definition of "unhappiness" was manifest (300.70; p. 252). Rooted in the work of the University of Iowa psychiatrists Nancy Andreasen and Janusz Bardach, the excessive concern with an "imaginary" defect came into its own in American psychiatry.[29] These patients only believed themselves to be "quite ugly" and were convinced that they "could be very attractive if some changes were made surgically" (673). Andreasen stressed that these patients were basically "content with their lives as they are but not with their appearance" (674). This category was introduced only as an example of atypical somatoform disorder.

By the 1994 edition of the *Diagnostic and Statistical Manual of Mental Disorders*, a full-scale discussion for the first time presented this diagnostic category in detail (300.7; pp. 466–69). It is a "preoccupation with a defect in appearance," which is "either excessive" or "imagined." The authors note that patients focus on specific aspects: "crooked" lip or "bumpy" nose but often "avoid describing their 'defects' in detail and may instead refer only to their general ugliness." Their preoccupations are self-described as "'intensely painful,' 'tormenting,' or 'devastating.'" The authors of DSM-IV evoke the use of the label "inferiority complex," which we shall discuss below, and present "dysmorphophobia" as rooted in "cultural concerns about physical appearance and the importance of proper physical self-presentation [which] may influence or amplify preoccupation about an imagined physical deformity. Preliminary evidence suggests that Body Dysmorphic Disorder is diag-

nosed with approximately equal frequency in women and men."
The underlying disorder is psychiatric; its symptoms take their
form from the cultural setting of the patient. By claiming the parity
of the sexes, however, the authors of DSM-IV place this disorder
beyond the world of aesthetic surgery, which is still gendered (at
least in 1994) as primarily female.

According to DSM-IV the diagnostic criteria for this syndrome
are preoccupation with an imagined defect; causing clinically significant stress or impairment of social, occupational, or other important areas of functioning; not accounted for by another mental
disorder (such as anorexia nervosa). These criteria could certainly
be applied to patients seeking aesthetic surgery for the amelioration of psychic "unhappiness." The boundary between the psychic
disorder that cannot be cured by surgery (a field beyond the com-
petency of the psychiatrist) and the physical anomaly that, if corrected, would cure "unhappiness" is made absolutely clear. It is of
little wonder that body dysmorphic disorder has come to be seen
as a form of obsessive-compulsive disorder that should be treated
by the most fashionable psychiatric therapy of the 1990s, psycho-
pharmacological intervention.[30] Yet there is still some discussion
of whether this syndrome, now labeled as a form of obsessive-
compulsive disorder because of the seeming efficacy of drug therapy (which makes the patients "happy"), does not still have a "psychotic" variant that is beyond the reach of drug treatment.[31] With
this question, the answer is given to those patients for whom happiness is not achieved through the suggested drug therapies.

Here we can see the movement to a psychiatric disorder for those
patients, who, as we shall note, aesthetic surgery is unsuccessful in
alleviating symptoms of unhappiness through allowing the patient
to "pass" as "normal." Yet the diagnostic criteria of DSM-IV are
keyed to the defect's being "imagined" or overvalued. These are
the same criteria that the aesthetic surgeons claim to be able to
correct so that the patients can pass as (in)visible. To operate or not
to operate? remains the question. The answer is often formulated
in terms of the mental health of the patient. Is the anxiety of the
patient "imagined" (and thus the patient is not a prime candidate
for surgery), or is it "real"? Here the complex boundary between
fields continues to play itself out.

Recently, an attempt has been made to create a popular diagnostic disorder to be called "BDD," abbreviating the DSM-diagnostic category of body dysmorphic disorder, to create a quickly quotable acronym with which to further compete with the expanding world of aesthetic surgery. Indeed, even Michael Jackson has been "diagnosed" as having the newest psychological disorder, "BDD," by a physician who, of course, never examined him. In July 1996 David Veale told the Association of European Psychiatrists conference in London that Jackson was a clear example of the condition: "He has had over 30 cosmetic surgery operations, his nose is reported to be crumbling, and his ex-wife Lisa Presley has said that he would never take off his make-up, even in bed."[32] Veale stated that the etiology of BDD lies in the fact that "the victims of the disorder have an over-developed aesthetic sense, meaning that they are more sensitive to beauty than most people and seek perfection in their own appearance. [Sounds like Jacques Joseph speaking!] BDD is most commonly diagnosed in people in their late 20s or early 30s and most victims have had the disorder for more than a decade. It affects both men and women." Here contemporary clinical psychiatry is still attempting to construct a "fashionable" illness (BDD to compete with BSE—mad cow disease) to compete with the increasingly ungendered world of aesthetic surgery.

The differential diagnosis to body dysmorphic disorder in DSM-IV is gender identity disorder (302.6; pp. 532–38), a category that plays a major role in discussions of transgender surgery.[33] If a patient focuses on any part of his or her body *besides* his or her primary or secondary sexual characteristics, one can diagnose body dysmorphic disorder; if the focus is *on* the primary or secondary sexual characteristics, then one can diagnose gender identity disorder. In contrast to body dysmorphic disorder, where the diagnosis precludes surgery, this diagnosis provides a psychological rationale for surgery.

The following are the diagnostic criteria for gender identity disorder: "A. Strong and persistent cross-gender identification (not merely a desire for any perceived cultural advantages of being the other sex). B. Persistent discomfort with his or her sex or sense of inappropriateness in the gender role of that sex: in boys, assertion that his penis or testes are disgusting or will disappear; in girls, assertion that she has or will grow a penis, or assertion that she does not want to grow breasts or menstruate. . . . C. This is not concurrent with a physical intersex condition (such as hermaphroditism). D. That it causes clinically significant distress or impairment in social, occupational, or other important areas of functioning." With this diagnosis the basis is presented for a specific form of aesthetic surgery—for the transformation or amputation of the primary and secondary characteristics and thus the alleviation of the psyche's pain.

The primary difference between diagnostic criteria (body dysmorphic disorder) that preclude surgery and those that advocate it (gender identity disorder) is the part(s) of the body on which the individual focuses. The meaning attributed to each and every body part is, of course, culturally and ideologically central to this distinction between the two categories. If you are "unhappy" with the imagined imperfection of your nose (as diagnosed by your psychiatrist) then you should be treated by psychotropic drugs; if you are "unhappy" with the imagined imperfection of your genitalia (as diagnosed by your psychiatrist) you should be treated with hormone therapy and surgery. The difference lies in the meaning attributed within psychoanalysis (and now clinical psychiatry) to the genitalia as a key to the psyche. The body maps the mind—but no longer by a nose. The movement between the restoration of function in society and the amelioration of "unhappiness" is often defined by the meanings attributed to specific body parts.

The clinical and phenomenological psychiatric response to the mind/body problem raised by aesthetic surgery was to develop a set of psychological criteria for the description of the internal life of the patients. Here the views of psychiatry and psychoanalysis were quite parallel. In claiming these patients for their own specialties, they denied the efficacy of surgery as psychotherapy. Surgeons such as Joseph needed to understand this rejection of the basic psychological explanation of the efficacy of his own field by adapting his model of surgery as psychotherapy even for cases of dysmorphophobia.

3. Ernst Kretschmer's Constitutional
Noses

The roots of the clinical definition of "unhappiness" with the body as formulated in clinical psychiatry of the nineteenth century lies in the science of race. Racial physiognomy in this context, as we have already seen, is defined to no little degree in the United States and Central Europe of the 1890s by the real and the metaphoric "Jew." Even more specifically, the part of the body that defines the Jew, at least in terms of public representations, is the nose. In Central European fantasy the Jew's nose was a permanent, visible sign of the difference of the Jew's body and psyche. It marked the essential nature of the Jew. Nothing, not acculturation and not baptism, could wipe away the taint of race. No matter how they changed their bodies, they still remained diseased and, therefore, dangerous Jews. This was marked on their physiognomy. Moses Hess (1812–1875), the German-Jewish revolutionary and political theorist commented in his *Rome and Jerusalem* (1862) that "even baptism will not redeem the German Jew from the nightmare of German Jew-hatred. The Germans hate less the religion of the Jews than their race, less their peculiar beliefs than their peculiar noses. . . . Jewish noses cannot be reformed, nor black, curly, Jewish hair be turned through baptism or combing into smooth hair. The Jewish race is a primal one, which had reproduced itself in its integrity despite climactic influences. . . . The Jewish type is indestructible."[1] The theme of the Jew's immutability was directly tied to arguments about the permanence of the negative features of the Jewish race.

On one count, Hess seemed to be wrong—the external appearance of the Jew did seem to be shifting without aesthetic surgery during the generations following civil emancipation at the beginning of the nineteenth century. His skin seemed to be getting whiter, his nose straighter, at least in his own estimation, though it could never get white enough or straight enough. In one of the most extraordinary representations of the mutable immutability of the Jew's body and psyche, the parodic novella "The Blood of the Walsungs" (1905), Thomas Mann (1875–1955) evokes an acculturated Jewish family in early-twentieth-century Berlin.[2] The father, a nouveau riche coal speculator from the eastern reaches of the German empire, collects first editions of the classics, but does so "gently rubbing his hands" and speaking in a "slightly plaintive way" (289). The mother, richly jeweled, is "small, ugly, prematurely aged, and shriveled as though by tropic sun" (290). She is badly (if expensively) dressed and coifed. She is the daughter of a "well-to-do tradesman" (and therefore mercantile by character) and reveals herself as Jewish by her speech, which was "interlarded with guttural words and phrases from the dialect of her childhood days" (294). If the mother is marked by her Jewish language (Mauscheln), the father is marked by disease—his is one of the illnesses of the rich, dyspepsia: "He suffered from a weakness of the solar plexus, that nerve center which lies at the pit of the stomach and may give rise to serious distress" (292). The four children of the family represent different types of Jews, but all are immutably Jewish in their seeming diversity. The oldest sibling Kunz, "a stunning tanned creature with curling lips and a killing scar"; Märit, "with a hooked nose, grey eyes like a falcon's and a bitter contemptuous mouth"; and the twins, Siglinde and Siegmund. Siegmund has a "sallow face." His "head is covered with thick black locks," and both share "the same slightly drooping nose, the same full lips lying softly together, the same prominent cheek-bones and black, bright eyes" (290). Later Siegmund carefully examines his face in the mirror: "Long he looked at each mark of his race: the slightly drooping nose, the full lips that rested so softly on each other; the high cheek bones, the thick black curling hair" (314). This description, including the shape of the nose, the form of the lips, and the "fact" that the Jew has "very heavy body and facial hair" (and is "extremely able in trade and business"), is a commonplace of the anti-Semitic ethnography of the age.[3] It is the physicality of the Jew that reveals his corrupt character—the twins end the tale by committing incest.

While emancipated Jews, at least in Western Europe, were no

longer believed to suffer from the disgusting skin diseases of poverty that had once marked their bodies, their nose could not be "reformed." The nose was a sign of the Jew's nature. George Jabet, writing as Eden Warwick, in his *Notes on Noses* (1848) asserted that the "Jewish, or Hawknose," is "very convex, and preserves its convexity like a bow, throughout the whole length from the eyes to the tip. It is thin and sharp." Shape also carried here a specific meaning: "It indicates considerable Shrewdness in worldly matters; a deep insight into character, and facility of turning that insight to profitable account."[4] Physicians, drawing on such analogies, speculated that the Jew's language, the very mirror of his psyche, was the result of the form of his nose. The language ascribed by Thomas Mann to the parents in his tale seems to magically reappear in the mouths of the children at the very close of this story. They begin to speak with a Yiddish accent. This was seen to be a sign of the physical immutability of the Jewish physiognomy. The young physician Bernhard Blechmann's rationale for the way the Jews spoke (*Mauscheln*), their inability to speak with other than a Jewish intonation, was that the "muscles, which are used for speaking and laughing are used inherently differently from those of Christians and that this use can be traced . . . to the great difference in their nose and chin."[5] The nose becomes one of the central loci of difference in defining the Jew.

It is the relationship between character and physiognomy that led Jewish social scientists, such as Joseph Jacobs (1854–1916), to confront the question of the "nostrility" of the Jews. He (and other Jewish scientists of the fin de siècle) saw that "the nose does contribute much toward producing the Jewish expression."[6] (These views continue well after the Shoah. Jacobs's mid-nineteenth-century images of "nostrility" are reproduced as "evidence" of Jewish physical difference in a respected textbook of physical anthropology in 1974.[7]) Jacobs puzzled about how to unmake the Jewish nose; how to alter the "nostrility" of the Jewish nose, a sign that does not even seem to vanish when the Jew is acculturated. Indeed, a detailed study of the anthropology of the "*Mischlinge* born to Jews and non-Jews" published in 1928 summarized the given view that there was a "Jew nose" and that this specific form of the nose was dominant in mixed marriages and was recognized to be a fixed, inherited sign of being Jewish.[8] In popular and medical imagery, the nose came to be the sign of the pathological Jewish character for Western Jews. The nose continued to have political significance. It was political within the constraints of the racial theory of the nineteenth century. "Big noses" cannot mate with "little noses." Even Edmond Rostand (1868–1918) in *Cyrano de Bergerac* (1897), which rejects the anti-Semitism of the Dreyfus affair, still imposes a racial theory onto the nose. In the play, "big noses," even noble noses, do not marry and procreate with "normal" noses, such as that of Roxanne. For in "mixing," the Jewish nose will always reveal itself, even if it is masked and unrecognized. Roland Barthes notes in his *Camera Lucida* that "Proust . . . said of Charles Haas (the model for Swann), according to George Painter, that he had a short, straight nose, but that old age had turned his skin to parchment, revealing the Jewish nose beneath."[9] The Jew within will always out.

Such views of Jewish malleability as written on their physiognomy was found among British Jews at the beginning of the twentieth century. The Anglo-Jewish artist Moysheh Oyved (1885–?) observed in 1927 that the Jewish nose may have been seen a sign of the decay of the Jew but that it was also a sign of the potential for Jewish reconstitution: "But my greatest joy was when I saw her giant nose, her awful 'pecker.' In her terribly large Jewish nose I saw the scaffold, the supporting-column, which the Creator of Heaven, Builder of Earth and Decorator of Spring had set down in the very middle of the face of a nation—a nation which is old, falling to pieces, but which is now being rebuilt anew."[10] With the advent of Nazi racial propaganda as part of daily experience, the meaning read into the Jewish nose during World War II came to heighten the idea that appearance was the key to difference. The concern about the continuation and integrity of the "group" is also written on the nose.

In *The Human Comedy* (1943), by William Saroyan (1908–1981), the central chapter in the education of the protagonist is called "A Speech on the Human Nose." In it, Homer Macauley addresses the centrality of the nose to human history: "The nose is perhaps the most ridiculous part of the human face. It has always been a source of embarrassment to the human race, and the Hittites probably beat up on everybody because their noses were so big and crooked."[11] Thus the notion of the "unhappy" psyche marked by the ugly nose that evokes disease is moved into the world of race and politics. Saroyan's intent was not to prove that difference is written on the face by the nose; rather, he stressed the universality of all human experience: "People all over the world have noses" (62). The racial implications of the nose are undercut in the following exchange:

> "Moses was in the Bible," Henry said.
> "Did he have a nose?" Joe said.
> "Sure he had a nose," Henry said.
> "All right, then," Joe said. "Why don't you say, 'Moses had a nose as big as most noses'? This is an ancient history class. Why don't you try to learn something once in a while? Moses —noses—ancient—history. Catch on?"
> Henry tried to catch on. "Moses noses," he said. "No, wait a minute. Moses' nose was a big nose."
> "Ah," Joe said, "You'll never learn anything. You'll die in the poorhouse. Moses had a nose as big as most noses!" (65–66)

Written at the height of Nazi attacks on the Jews, Saroyan's novel is a novel about war, death, and tolerance as seen from small-town California from the perspective of its Armenian author. In the various systems of physiognomy that dominated popular consciousness during the late nineteenth and early twentieth centuries bad character was associated with big noses. Both were seen in the image of the Jew. This exchange evokes all of the claims for a difference written on the face, a difference that marks the superior from the inferior and ironically destroys them.

It is not merely that second- and third-generation descendants of Eastern European Jewish immigrants do not "look" like their grandparents, but that they "look" American, having "passed on" their new features in a Lamarckian manner. This seemed quite parallel to the physical acculturation claimed for the Jews of Germany by Virchow and for turn-of-the-century Eastern European Jews by Boas. This fantasy, like the images of Virchow and Boas, demand the malleability of the Jewish body spontaneously to fit the idealized aesthetic model of "American" culture. The writer and director Philip Dunne commented on the fantasy of physical acculturation of Jews in Southern California during the twentieth century:

You could even see the physical change in the family in the second generation—not resembling the first generation at all. Of course, this is true all across the country, but it is particularly noticeable in people who come out of very poor families. . . . One dear friend and colleague of mine was a product of a Lower East Side slum. He was desperately poor. And he grew up a rickety, tiny man who had obviously suffered as a child. At school, he told me, the goyim would scream at him. Growing up in California, his two sons were tall, tanned, and blond. Both excelled academically and in athletics. One became a military officer, the other a physicist. They were California kids. Not only American but Californian.[12]

One is never aware of the difference of one's body—whether it is real or constructed—until one learns about it by seeing the Other. This difference is associated with the exotic and the distanced, as the contemporary British novelist Julian Barnes (1946-) has his protagonist note about one of his Jewish friends:

Toni far outclassed me in rootlessness. His parents were Polish Jews and, though we didn't actually know it for certain, we were practically sure that they had escaped from the Warsaw ghetto at the very last minute. This gave Toni the flash foreign name of Barbarowski, two languages, three cultures, and a sense (he assured me) of atavistic wrench: in short, real class. He looked an exile, too: swarthy, bulbous-nosed, thick-lipped, disarmingly short, energetic and hairy; he even had to shave every day.[13]

Barnes romanticizes all of the negative images associated with the Jew but still associates them with the physical difference of the Jew. This is not all that far from the nineteenth-century aspect of Charles Dickens's Fagin (with his "villainous and repulsive face") or George du Maurier's Svengali (whose "Jewish aspect [was] well featured but sinister"). It is associated with the difference and the distance of the Jew in British society.[14] The actual acculturation of the Jew into British society could in no way disguise the Jew's visibility.

We can see this operation in effect once again in the writings of Walter Lippmann (1889–1974), one of the leading Jewish American intellectuals of the first half of the twentieth century, who commented in the late 1920s that:

> the rich and vulgar and pretentious Jews of our big American cities are perhaps the greatest misfortune that has ever befallen the Jewish people. They are the fountain of anti-Semitism. When they rush about in super automobiles, bejeweled and furred and painted and overbarbered, when they build themselves French chateaux and Italian palazzi, they stir up the latent hatred against crude wealth in the hands of shallow people; and that hatred diffuses itself.[15]

The Jew remains a Jew even when disguised. It is in the Jew's "painted and overbarbered" essence. One cannot hide—nose job or no nose job—from the lessons of race, and the Jew is the most aware of this. Lippmann creates in his mind's eye the image of his antithesis, the "bad" Jew to his "good" Jew. And this Jew is just as visible as he believes himself to be (in)visible. Lippmann, in his Wall Street suit and carefully controlled manners and appearance, looks just like everyone else, or so he hopes. But there is no hiding from the fact of a constructed difference. There is no mask, no operation, no refuge.

In the psychological theory of the early twentieth century the argument that linked the physical type to the character in the most direct way was formulated by Ernst Kretschmer. His theory of constitutional types argued against transformation as a model. This reaction to the Darwinian view of the mutability of form is best captured in the debates around the attempt in the 1920s to apply the body-type thesis of Ernst Kretschmer to racial biology.[16] Kretschmer's three body types (asthenic, athletic, pyknic) had been associated with specific forms of psychological character. Given the general assessment that there was a close correlation between race and character, it was not too long before this leap was made. Ludwig Stern-Piper, in a lecture at the 1922 Southwest German Psychiatric Conference, took the three body types outlined by Kretschmer and claimed that his constitutional types were the basic racial types.[17] Kretschmer responded in the next issue.[18] He saw the existence of all three body types in all races; indeed he saw a certain contradiction between the very concept of "racial" types and body types. Stern-Piper continued the argument, stressing the inherent racial makeup of each individual and the links between body type, illness, and race.[19] This debate was joined by clinicians such as the Munich physician Moses Julius Gutmann (1894–?), who attempted to correlate Kretschmer's notion of constitutional types with specific mental illnesses. The so-called predominance among Jews, he notes, of the asthenic body type of a long, lanky body, suggested to him that they would be particularly subject to schizophrenia, but in his own clinical work he found a predominance of manic-depressive psychosis among Jews.[20] It is clear from examples such as this that the way the Jew looks, like the way the criminal looks, was considered scientific evidence of the Jew's inherently pathological condition.

Constitutional debates also hung on a nose. On March 7, 1913, Julius Tandler (1869–1936), the Jewish professor of anatomy and Viennese city councilor, had addressed the German Society for Racial Hygiene (that is, Eugenics).[21] Tandler illustrated his distinction between constitution and race with a specific example. While some, he argues, see the shape of the nose as a constitutional sign, he sees it as racial. He observed that individuals with a "Jewish nose" (*Hakennase*) are born with a small, flat nose and the development of the Jewish nose takes place only at puberty (21). Following the belief of Enlightenment physiology, Tandler asserts that the universal nose is formed in the earliest stages of fetal development; the racial nose appears as the individual matures and becomes identified as a part of the race. Here Tandler seems to exclude the "exterior" presentation of the body, which might not reflect the internal habitus of the individual, that is, one may look different from what one truly is.

Following Kretschmer, Tandler divides all individuals into three types based on musculature and muscle tone: the hypertonic, the normal-tonic, and the hypotonic. Note that this typology is not just physical but also psychological; thus Botticelli is, for Tandler, the painter of the hypotonic, and Michelangelo the painter of the hypertonic (17–18). He goes further to suggest that this is because they themselves were hypo- or hypertonic: "Great artists as rigidly formed individuals cannot transcend their own muscle tone and they paint this. If they are hypotonic [they paint] only hypotonic individuals, if they are hypertonic, only hypertonic individuals" (17). The creative artist's manner of seeing the world is limited by habitus: epistemology is thus a reflex of biology, and by extension, to bring this argument back to the nose, no surgery on the nose can change the way one sees the world.

The Jewish body can seem to be changed through acculturation, but adaptability becomes merely a further sign of the immutability of racial constitution. Werner Sombart (1863–1941), in *The Jews and Modern Capitalism* (1911), provided a clear image of the Jewish body as a sign of its adaptability (as a sign of its inherent immutability). For Sombart it is the very fact that the Jew is always able to change that marks the Jew's character: "He is a German where he wants to be German, and Italian if that suits him better. He does everything and dabbles in everything, and with success. He can be a pure Magyar in Hungary, he can belong to the Irredenta in Italy, and be an anti-Semite in France (Drumont!)." So the political and economic mutability of the Jew is paralleled by the physical ability of the Jew's body to change.

> The driving power in Jewish adaptability is of course the idea of a purpose, or a goal, as the end of all things. Once the Jew has made up his mind what line he will follow, the rest is comparatively easy, and his mobility only makes his success more sure. How mobile the Jew can be is positively astounding. He is able to give himself the personal appearance he most desires. . . . The best illustrations may be drawn from the United States, where the Jew of the second or third generation is with more difficulty distinguished from the non-Jew. You can tell the German after no matter how many generations; so with the Irish, the Swede, the Slav. But the Jew, in so far as his racial features allow it, has been successful in imitating the Yankee type, especially in regard to outward marks such as clothing, bearing and the peculiar method of hairdressing.[22]

Sombart's view is echoed in the bodybuilding literature of the turn of the century. The Jew's new body, whether acquired through surgery or through exercise, is drawn into question. "The well-educated person who is only an imitator taking his opinions and his mannerisms from others; the vain parodic attempts of the parvenu, the master-butcher, the tailor's apprentice, the baron Kohns of this world to align themselves in excellence of mind and body," according to Sombart, with members of a healthy race and a healthy class.[23] This sense of spontaneous physical transformation in the age of aesthetic surgery suggests that while the Jew is chameleon-like there are some subliminal signs that signal the Jew, so that complete "passing" is impossible. Can total physical transformation become a reality? The response to this question forms the leitmotif for the representation and self-representation of the Jew in the culture of late-nineteenth-century Europe.

Ironically, the more Jews in Germany and Austria at the fin de siècle began to look like their non-Jewish contemporaries, the more they sensed themselves as different and were so considered. As Joseph Jacobs (1854–1916), the Anglo-Jewish social scientist, noted, "it is some quality which stamps their features as distinctly Jewish. This is confirmed by the interesting fact that Jews who mix much with the outer world seem to lose their Jewish quality. This was the case with Karl Marx."[24] Yet, as we know, it was precisely those Jews who were the most assimilated, who were passing, who feared that their visibility as Jews could come to the fore. It was they who most feared being seen as bearing that disease, Jewishness, that the mid-nineteenth-century German-Jewish poet Heinrich Heine (1797–1856) said the Jews brought from Egypt. For Heine, too, in his memorial to the German-Jewish writer Ludwig Börne, it is the body, specifically the "long nose which is a type of uniform, by which the King-God Jehovah recognizes his old retainers, even if they had deserted."[25] Conversion of the soul is not an answer to this immutable marking of the Jewish body and the Jewish soul; the transformation of the body through surgery may well be the parallel to conversion in secular society.

In late-nineteenth-century thought those aspects of the body that marked one as Jewish were associated with specific qualities of mind and character. For example, the famed German artist and poet Wilhelm Busch (1832–1908), in his best known work *Pious Helene* (1872), read the Jew's usurious soul into the image of the Jew's body:

> Und der Jud mit krummer Ferse
> Krummer Nas' und krummer Hos',

> Schlängelt sich zur hohen Börse
> Tiefverderbt und seelenlos!
> [And the Hebrew, sly and craven,
> Round of shoulder, nose, and knee,
> Slinks to the Exchange, unshaven
> And intent on usury.][26]

The nose is not merely a sign of the difference and illness of the body, but also of the social illness represented by the Jew in German society, an illness of the body politic. The Jew's nose comes to represent the Jew's permanently sick soul.[27]

Constitution, the inherent structure of the body, continues to be understood as mirroring character; thus it is not at all surprising that as late as the 1970s, aesthetic surgery comes to be understood as "somatopsychic therapy." The Hungarian physician Alfred Berndorfer uses the label "organopsychic" rather than somatopsychic, but means much the same thing. The surgeon is operating as much on the psyche as on the body. For Berndorfer this may be seen in terms of theories of constitution: "Knowing the type of constitution and face, a person may form himself or let his features be changed accordingly. The psychic problem has to be known by every physician who is engaged in aesthetic surgery."[28] The problem for the aesthetic surgeon is the complex claim that surgery on the body will "cure" the psyche, not only of its "unhappiness," but of the causes of that unhappiness, its racial difference. The background to such views must be sought in the Enlightenment. The more you change, the more you remain the same.

The very theory that supported the view that the Jew's damaged psyche could be repaired was itself contested. If constitutional arguments were right, then there was a fixed body and a fixed character; for example, Hans Blüher (1888–1955) dismisses "the Jew Freud" and his notion of psychosomatic correlates, which represent only the most modern version of corrosive Jewish thought.[29] Here his views paralleled those of Enrico Morselli. These views of the mind-body relationship, according to anti-Semitic thinkers at the beginning of the century, are to be found already in the *Ethics* of Benedictus de Spinoza (1632–1677), whom they see as arguing for the identity of body and spirit. For Spinoza, as for Freud, when something occurs in the body it is because it occurs in the spirit:

"Wherever spirit is there is also body. Every idea has a corporeal correlate" (25). The identity of mind and body, a central theme in Joseph's understanding of his patients, is merely a Jewish "trick" to get Aryans to believe that their "Geist" (spirit) and their bodies are crassly, materialistically linked. What seems to be a "neutral" model of argumentation, the model of psychosomatic and somato-psychic illness, is revealed as "Jewish." Such views impact on the Jewish physician, such as Sigmund Freud, as well as his patients and often these were interchangeable.

4. Sigmund Freud's Nose Job

Aesthetic surgery began in the operating theaters of New York, Vienna, and Berlin in the 1880s through the development of procedures altering the shapes of noses. Surgery on the nose would change the "unhappy" state of the psyche, according to this view. In addition to the aesthetic surgeons, there were at least two other Jewish physicians in fin de siècle Europe who were preoccupied with the nose and who went a step further to argue that there is a direct relationship between the "nose" and the "genitalia." And through the genitalia there was a further link to the psyche. For them, too, if you operated on the nose, you could directly alter the "unhappiness" of your patient.

For the Berlin otorhinolaryngologist Wilhelm Fliess (1858–1928) and his Viennese collaborator, the neurologist Sigmund Freud, the nose came to serve as a sign of universal development rather than as a specific sign of an "inferior" racial identity.[1] The nose was the developmental analogy to the genitalia. Evolving embryologically at the same stage, there was a shared relationship between the tissue of the nose and that of the genitalia. For Fliess and Freud, this was true of all human beings, not only Jews. It followed that one cure for sexual dysfunction and hysteria, according to Fliess, was to operate on the nose and that he regularly did.

Fliess's theories reflect a fascination with the link between human anatomy and psychology. His work centered on the relationship between the periodic cycle (which he claimed to discern in men and women) as well as the relationship between the anatomy of the genitalia and that of the nose. Fliess's surgical interventions focused on the nose and its relationship to the female menstrual cycle. He observed a swelling of the turbinate bone of the nose during menstruation and claimed to have discovered "genital spots" on the inside of the nose.

In 1897 he evolved a theory about the relationship between menstruation and periodicity. While the menstrual cycle was twenty-eight days; other cycles of twenty-three days were also present. These views were supported within mainstream medicine of the late nineteenth century, as in the work of Moriz Benedikt (1835–1920) in Vienna and John Nolan Mackenzie (1853–1925) at Johns Hopkins.[2] Fliess's theories, based on the best of late-nineteenth-century endocrinological and neurological theory, appeared to the late-nineteenth-century physician as seriously scientific. In a detailed account of "the relation between the nose and the sexual apparatus," an anonymous author in the *Boston Medical and Surgical Journal* for 1898 summarized both Mackenzie's and Fliess's work in detail.[3] Commenting on Fliess, the essay states that "we may be able in future to do away with one of our two common sources of peripheral irritation and treat all of our patients through the nose . . . by cocainization and cauterizing these spots." Fascinating as this may seem from our contemporary viewpoint, this is not the central point. More important is the way the essay ends with the following statement: "And if we can also recover the lost art of the ancients, and add to our requirements the diagnosis of the sexual condition of those we meet by the size and shape of the nose and mouth and neck we shall add greatly to the chastity of the race; for who would dare to transgress if his transgression were to be written on his face?" The reading (and treating) of the nose assures the health of the race through the avoidance of sexual infection, miscegenation, and perversion. Fliess's surgical procedures fulfilled a function for him, as well as for Sigmund Freud, in creating a sense of how surgical interventions in the body could cure the disturbances of the psyche. Others read them as the ability to extirpate the foreign and diseased from the body politic.

Fliess's patients did not make up a cross section of society. Of the 156 cases he records (some from the medical literature of the time), only a dozen were men.[4] All of the rest were women, who were operated upon for numerous complaints, primarily psychological ones. Fliess treated a wide range of mental illnesses, including hysteria, through the extensive use of cocaine, but he also applied acid to the internal structures of the nasal passages or surgically removed them.

This association of the nose with the genitalia was not perceived only as a "woman's problem" in the popular mind. The central sign of male periodicity for Fliess (and for Freud) was male menstruation.[5] Its representation, according to Freud in his July 20, 1897, letter to Fliess, was an "occasional bloody nasal secretion."[6] Later, in his letter of October 15, 1897, Freud traces the implications of male menstruation for himself as well as (one assumes) for Fliess:

> My self-analysis is in fact the most essential thing I have at present and promises to become of the greatest value to me if it reaches its end. In the middle of it, it suddenly ceased for three days, during which I had the feeling of being tied up inside (which patients complain of so much), and I was really disconsolate until I found that these same three days (twenty-eight days ago) were the bearers of identical somatic phenomena. Actually only two bad days with a remission in between. From this one should draw the conclusion that the female period is not conducive to work. Punctually on the fourth day, it started again. Naturally, the pause also had another determinant—the resistance to something surprisingly new. Since then I have been once again intensely preoccupied [with it], mentally fresh, though afflicted with all sorts of minor disturbances that come from the content of the analysis.[7]

There is a lively nineteenth-century medical literature on this topic, by writers such as F. A. Forel and W. D. Halliburton, as well as a fascination with this question in regard to the problem of hermaphroditism as a sign of bisexuality.[8] Professor Paul Albrecht in Hamburg argued for the existence of "male menstruation," which was periodic and which mimicked the menstrual cycle of the female through the release of white corpuscles into the urine.[9] In the writing of the sexologist Paul Näcke (1851–1913), there was a detailed discussion of the question of "male menstruation" and its relationship to the problem of periodicity.[10] Näcke cited among others Havelock Ellis (1859–1939) who had been collecting material on this question for years.

With the rise of modern sexology at the close of the nineteenth century, especially in the writings of Magnus Hirschfeld (1868–1935), male menstruation came to hold a very special place in the "proofs" for the continuum between male and female sexuality and for the potential for transgender surgery.[11] The hermaphrodite, the male who menstruated, became one of the central focuses of Hirschfeld's work. But all of this new "science" that used the existence of male menstruation still drew on the image of the marginality of those males who menstruated and thus pointed toward a much more ancient tradition.

But it was Fliess's skill (or lack of it) as a surgeon that saw the realization of his theories concerning the relationship between the nose and human sexuality. As is the case today, "nose" doctors were also surgeons. His surgical ineptitude almost killed Freud's patient Emma Eckstein in late February 1895. He had operated on her nose intranasally to "cure" her of her hysteria but caused massive bleeding and infection. Fliess operated on Freud's nose during the same stay in Vienna in which he operated on Emma Eckstein. The operation on Eckstein was seriously botched by Fliess, who left "half a meter of gauze" in the nasal passage following the procedure. Freud was overwhelmed by the sudden downward course of his patient but could not turn to Fliess who had in the meantime returned to Berlin.

On March 4, 1895, Freud wrote to Fliess to tell him what had transpired.[12] Fearing for his patient's life he called in Robert Gersuny (1844–1924) for a consultation. Gersuny was one of the major figures in aesthetic surgery in Vienna. He had been Theodor Billroth's student in the field of surgery and was appointed by him to head the surgical department of his hospital, the Rudolfinerhaus, in 1888.[13] He had developed the first "island flap" in 1887, in repairing with subcutaneous tissues the floor of the mouth of a young woman suffering from cancer. But it was as the innovator of paraffin injections to rebuild the face that he would become as infamous as Fliess. For his procedures, too, caused facial deformations and death as the paraffin spread under the skin.

Gersuny was known as the "greatest diagnostician" of his day.[14] Freud's calling upon Gersuny was not only bringing a notable surgeon in on his case, but one who subscribed to the basic somatopsychological theories as did Fliess. The relationship between the

surgeon and the patient becomes for Gersuny analogous to that between the psychoanalyst and the analysand.[15] He wrote that "the
patient should first be allowed to narrate without interruption the
history of his complaint before any questions are put to him" (22).
Doctors should take the psychological complaints of their patients
seriously. For the "first thing a sick person desires is to get rid of
his disagreeable sensations" (26). Gersuny also shared Freud's aesthetic taste. Freud notes proudly that upon entering his surgery,
Gersuny "admired an etching of the *Isle of the Dead* by [Arnold]
Böcklin" (113–14). Aesthetics remains part of what makes a good
academic surgeon truly part of his culture.

On March 8, 1895, Gersuny is again called in to consult with
Freud about Eckstein. Later that day Gersuny is unavailable when
Eckstein continues to bleed and Freud asks his old friend, the otorhinolaryngologist Ignaz Rosanes to examine the patient, and it
is he who discovers the forgotten gauze. In Freud's letter reporting this to Fliess, it is also clear that Gersuny has performed some
type of surgical procedure on Eckstein in the recent past (116). On
March 13 Gersuny operates on Eckstein again to stanch the bleeding (121).

All the procedures on the nose (carried out on Eckstein as well
as Freud) attempted to cure the mind through intervention in the
body. It was a surgical cure of the psyche and that becomes the
thrust of Freud's halfhearted attempt to assuage Fliess. He wrote to
him, "For me you remain the physician, the type of man into whose
hands one confidently puts one's life and that of one's family—even
if Gersuny should have the same opinion of your skills as *Weil*"
(125). The Viennese internist Moriz Weil wrote about the botched
Eckstein affair in a public essay in 1897: "We have achieved the
insight that *it is less important to discover new operations and
new methods of operating than to search for ways and methods to
avoid operations.*"[16] This is precisely the opposite of the desire of
both doctors and patients involved in aesthetic surgery and Fliess's
"nasal interventions." They all need new procedures to be able to
intervene in ways that (they believed) no one had yet undertaken.
Many of their contemporaries saw this as a form of quackery.

Much later Sigmund Freud stated that if psychoanalysis was to
be taken seriously as a therapeutic system it had to rid itself of

the label of "quackery." Many of the early attacks on psychoanalysis labeled it as pseudoreligious quackery. When this came to be tested in a court of law in 1926, Freud wrote a long essay titled "Psychoanalysis and Quackery." (It has come into the psychoanalytic literature under the more neutral title, "The Question of Lay Analysis.") In it he defended not only Theodor Reik (1888–1969) against the attack of being a lay person practicing medicine without adequate medical training, but psychoanalysis as a true form of therapy. His definition of quackery is striking. For Freud, "honesty compels [him] to admit that the activity of an untrained analyst does less harm to his patients than that of an unskilled surgeon."[17] But what sort of surgeon is it that Freud has in mind: "All this is undesirable, but it bears no comparison with the dangers that threaten from the knife of a surgical quack." The "surgical quack" is the surgeon who does harm, who almost kills his patient. Here the case of Fliess becomes the litmus test for the "quack." It is the rhinological surgeon, whose work was to complement psychoanalysis, but now is clearly much more dangerous to the health and well-being of the patient than the work of the psychoanalyst. Not the aesthetic surgeon, but Fliess, is the person Freud has in mind, and yet the claims that one could cure the psyche by operating on the body link the two in powerful ways.

The quack surgeon operated on the nose and claimed he was operating on the psyche through magically altering the genitalia. It was not merely that in turn-of-the-century Europe there was an association between the genitalia and the nose; there was, and had long been, a direct relationship drawn in popular and medical thought between the size of the nose and that of the penis. Ovid wrote, as we have quoted from Wilhelm Stekel, "Noscitur e naso quanta sit hast viro." The link between the Jew's sexuality, his circumcised (castrated) penis, and his nose was a similarly well-established one at century's end, but here the traditional pattern was reversed.[18] The specific shape of the Jew's nose indicated the damaged nature, the shortened form, of his penis. The traditional positive association between the size of the nose and that of the male genitalia was reversed and this reversal was made a pathological sign.[19] This evocation of the size of the nose and the penis was a measure of the libidinous nature of the Jews. As often quoted as the passage from Ovid, was the well-known passage from Cornelius Tacitus (certainly no friend of the Jews): "Separati epulis discreti cubilibus, proiectissima ad libidinem gens, alienarum concubitu abstinent" (*Historia* V, 1, 5). Historically, this association used the image of the "foëtor judaicus," the stench attributed to the Jews, and the low status of the aesthetics of smell as representing Jewish difference.[20] The association between the Jewish nose and the circumcised penis, as signs of Jewish difference, was made in the crudest and most revolting manner during the 1880s.

In the streets of Berlin and Vienna, in penny-papers or on the newly installed "Litfassäulen," or advertising columns, caricatures of Jews could be seen.[21] An image of the essential Jew, little "Mr. Kohn," showed him drowned, only his nose and huge, oversized feet showing above the waterline.[22] These extraordinary caricatures stressed one central aspect of the physiognomy of the Jewish male, his nose, which represented that hidden sign of his sexual difference, his circumcised penis. The Jews' sign of sexual difference, their sexual selectivity, as an indicator of their identity was, as Friedrich Nietzsche strikingly observed in *Beyond Good and Evil*, the focus of the Germans' fear of the superficiality of their recently created national identity.[23] This fear was represented in caricatures by the elongated nose. It also permeated the scientific discussions of the time. In the "anatomical-anthropological" study of the nose (1893) by Viennese anatomist, Oskar Hovorka (1866–1930), the form of the nose is seen as a sign of negative racial difference, as well as a sign of the "idiot and the insane."[24] Look at the nose of the Other and you will see the basic sign of the atavism. Thus, when Wilhelm Fliess attempted to alter the pathology of the genitalia by operating on the nose, at a point in time when national identity was extremely unsure of itself and scapegoats easy to find, he joined the Enlightenment universalistic theory to the German biology of race. Fliess's desire was to make this into a quality of all human beings, male and female, Jew and Aryan, not merely of Jewish males. He succeeded in generating an image of the woman as the sufferer from the pathologies of the nose that was equivalent to the general cultural view of the Jewish male.

Fliess's goal—like that of so many others of the time—was to alter the Jewish body so that the Jew could become (in)visible.

Some Jews, such as the Berlin literary critic Ludwig Geiger (1848–1919), rebelled against this desire for a Jewish invisibility: "If one desires assimilation—and that can only mean becoming German in morals, language, actions, feelings—one needs neither mixed marriages nor baptism. No serious person would suggest an assimilation which demanded that all Jews had straight noses and blond hair."[25] In arguing the point this way Geiger was reacting to precisely those pressures that caused Jews to dye their hair and "bob" their noses. Geiger implies that the changes are primarily for cosmetic purposes, vanity's sake. What he pointedly avoids discussing is that they were actually meant to "cure" the disease of Jewishness, the anxiety of being seen as a Jew. Being seen as a Jew meant being persecuted, attacked, and harassed. The "cure" for this was the actual alteration of the body. The Jewish mind, which German culture saw as different from that of the Aryan, is afflicted by its sense of its own difference. To cure the Jew's mind and make him "happy," Joseph and Fliess had to operate on the Jew's nose. Fliess's operation demanded the universality of all human experience without any differences in racial terms; Joseph's procedures effaced the markers of Jewish difference. Both aimed to make the Jew's psyche happier by altering the Jew's body.

5. Sigmund Freud's Castration Anxiety

The core argument concerning aesthetic surgery was shaped within the crucible of theories of the racial aesthetic and the aesthetic of the healthy body. It was formulated by surgeons who were evolving procedures that altered the body—and made the patient "happy." Theirs was, as we have seen, a pragmatic understanding of the psychology of their patients, a psychology without the complications of an unconscious. The conscious mind (or perhaps one could say, the self-conscious mind) that they promulgated had not changed much since the Renaissance in spite of the dominance of Cartesian dualism from the seventeenth century to the Enlightenment. It was a mind in which all events took place in the conscious present, and that presentism was defined in terms of the construction of "in" groups and "out" groups. For Jews and blacks and syphilitics, according to the medical mythmaking of the late nineteenth century, also existed only in the present moment; and their illnesses, the illnesses of ugliness, were the cause of their unhappiness. But what was healthy and what was diseased, what caused unhappiness and what was the cure that brought happiness? Much of the concern of aesthetic surgery focused on what must be cured—the mind or the body? Thus all of the early arguments about the efficacy of aesthetic surgery rest on arguments about the relationship between mind and body, and these in turn are best exemplified by the examples taken from the world of racial science. Race more than any other category provided a rationale and a model for "passing" in the world of nineteenth-century surgeons and was closely related to the representation of healthy and unhealthy bodies and character in the work of contemporary aesthetic surgeons.

How such case material actually "shaped" the psychological argument as well as how it was formed by that argument can be seen in another account of the severe psychological damage done by the internalization of this sense of the "Jewish nose." It is not from the surgical literature but from the psychoanalytic literature of the early twentieth century. We must remember that following Fliess's botched attempt to operate on Freud's patient Emma Eckstein (and Freud himself) in 1895, Freud broke with the "trauma theory." He stopped, according to his own statement, believing that real life events, such as child seduction and physical trauma, were at the core of mental illness. He no longer believed his neurotics and he abandoned the materialist theories of Fliess, who saw the body itself as the means of accessing the psyche. After 1896, he no longer believed one could alter the psyche by operating on the body. Freud stopped seeing the outside to the body as a means of judging the internal workings of the psyche and began to focus on the invisible and unseeable aspects of the psyche. He now saw the fantasy as the source for the types of physical ailments that manifested themselves in sexual dysfunction and hysteria.

By the beginning of the twentieth century, aesthetic surgery had firmly established itself in Vienna in the presence of Theodor Billroth and his student, the aesthetic surgeon Robert Gersuny, who attempted to rescue Emma Eckstein. Freud, too, was confronted with the implied psychology of the aesthetic surgeons, who argued, much as Fliess had, that operating on the body would ameliorate the psyche. We have one case of Freud's response to aesthetic surgery. It comes from the case file of his first biographer and one of the first psychoanalysts, the Viennese-Jewish physician Fritz Wittels (1880–1950). At the meeting of the Viennese Psychoanalytic Society on December 9, 1908, Wittels recounted a case of a patient who had come to him specifically because of the publication of his polemical work on baptized Jews—Jews who were trying to pass as Christians.[1] Wittels saw such conversions as a form of insanity. "Passing" was an impossibility for the medical mind of the turn of the century, because it meant imagining oneself as inherently different in biological terms. This was considered to be a form of psychosis.

Wittels presented the case of a young man of about thirty who suffered from "anti-Semitic persecution, for which he held his inconspicuously Semitic nose responsible. The patient planned to have the shape of his nose changed by plastic surgery."[2] Wittels, in turn, attempted to persuade him that his anxiety about his (inconspicuous but clearly Semitic!) nose was merely a displacement for anxiety about his sexual identity: "This the patient declared to be a good joke." The evident error for Wittels's suggestions does not occur to Wittels. If a patient came to him expressly because of his writing about the neurosis of conversion and wished to have his nose rebuilt to hide his Jewishness, then the question of his own "paranoid" relationship to his own circumcised penis, that (in)visible but omnipresent sign of the male's Jewishness, is self-evident to the patient.

Freud picked up on this argument directly and noted that "the man is evidently unhappy about being a Jew and wants to be baptized." In 1895 unhappiness is Freud's pessimistic label for the quality of normal daily life and yet here he makes the now pathological unhappiness of the patient contingent on something quite apart from the internal mechanisms of the psyche. He places it in the society in which he dwells and sees it as an artifact of the superego, that part of the psyche that monitors and is monitored by the values and laws of the world in which the individual dwells. Central to the comments of Wittels and Freud is the powerful assumption that it is the internal life of the patient that makes his external reality the focus of his "unhappiness." It is the mind that makes the body the locus of its neurosis.

But "passing" for this patient did not mean simply denying his Jewish identity: "At this point Wittels remarks that the patient is an ardent Jew. Nevertheless, he does not undergo baptism. In this fact lies the conflict that has absorbed the meaning of other conflicts." To be a Jew and to be so intensely fixated on the public visibility of that identity is to be ill. This obsession is actually stressed by Wittels's comment on the "inconspicuous" yet clearly "Semitic" nature of his patient's nose. One assumes that this would be a self-description of Wittels's own physiognomy. Baptism is impossible because it can only "cure" the soul, not reform the body. It cannot make the Jewish nose invisible.

Wittels then revealed the name of the patient to the group and Freud recognized from the name that the patient's father was an engaged Zionist. He then read the desire to unmake himself as a Jew as a sign of the rejection of the father. Freud, however, did not comment on the link between a strong Jewish identity and the rejection of the visibility that that identity entailed. There was a real sense in Freud's comment that the Jewish body, represented by the skin or the nose, could never truly be changed. It was a permanent, constitutional fixture, forever reflecting the Jew's racial identity. Altering the Jew's external form may have provided a wider margin in which the Jew could "pass," but the Jew could never be truly at peace with the sense of his or her invisibility. The unhappiness that Freud finds in the patient and feels constrained to redefine in terms of psychic mechanisms (anxiety about identifying with the father) is precisely the same unhappiness that the aesthetic surgeons of Freud's day sought to eliminate through their procedures.

The image of the Jewish body as an unchangeable one and one that leads in its visibility to psychopathology appears in one further discussion in which Wittels took part. On January 12, 1910, Wittels presented his infamous account of the "neurosis" of his contemporary, the "hunch-backed" Viennese writer and lecturer, Karl Kraus (1874–1936). Kraus's corrosive wit and antipsychoanalytic position were credited to his bodily deformity: "Kraus is a misshapen man, as was Voltaire, and as court jesters are described as having been. Mockery seems to be linked with physical deformity, and in that way to be suitable as a special domain of the Jews, in accordance with a remark Freud made in the analysis of the phobia of a five-year-old boy. [Little Hans] (Castration complex—circumcision.)" (2: 387). Wittels's reference to Freud's case of "Little Hans" is a complex one.

Freud had noted that the anxiety about castration in the child may well have been tied to the actual act of ritual circumcision that he had undergone. In the 1909 case of the Jewish child who is called "Little Hans," Freud paraphrases the child's argument: "Could it be that living beings really exist which did not possess widdlers? If so, it would no longer be so incredible that they could take his own widdler away, and, as it were, make him into a woman!"[3] This is linked to the common charge at the turn of the century, that Jews have no claim on true "wit," only destructive mockery. This is central to the representation of the Jew by Otto

Weininger (1880–1903) in his 1903 *Sex and Character*. As Freud writes in his study of "Little Hans":

> The castration complex is the deepest root of anti-Semitism; for even in the nursery little boys hear that a Jew has something cut off his penis—a piece of his penis, they think—and this gives them a right to despise Jews. And there is no stronger unconscious root for the sense of superiority over women. Weininger (the young philosopher who, highly gifted but sexually deranged, committed suicide after producing his remarkable book, *Geschlecht und Charakter* [*Sex and Character*, 1903]), in a chapter that attracted much attention, treated Jews and women with equal hostility and overwhelmed them with the same insults. Being neurotic, Weininger was completely under the sway of his infantile complexes; and from that standpoint what is common to Jews and women is their relation to the castration complex.[4]

In his study of the case of "Little Hans," Freud read the actual alteration of the body, the circumcision of the child, as marking the child's psyche through his sense of the mutability of his body. Castration anxiety is the anxiety about losing the penis and being made into something different and less whole. To this statement Freud appends a long footnote that relates the anxiety about castration to the nature of anti-Semitism.

It is important to follow Freud's stated train of thought: if—says the child—I can be circumcised and made into a Jew, can I not also be castrated and be made into a woman? The child has a "real" sense of castration anxiety, somewhere between that of the idealized types of the "little girl" who believes herself to have been castrated and the "little boy" who fears being castrated. The anxiety about bodily difference is a social phenomenon that Freud makes the source of "unhappiness." Circumcision, the alteration of the body, creates the conditions where "unhappiness" is exaggerated.

Given the role that Freud has circumcision play in the psychic life of the child, it is clear that Freud did not advocate that the child be raised as anything but a Jew. Neither conversion nor decircumcision could truly alter the Jewishness of his patient. In a letter to Max Graf, the father of "Little Hans," Freud argued that having

Graf's son baptized would not change his essential "Jewishness": "If you do not let your son grow up as a Jew, you will deprive him of those sources of energy which cannot be replaced by anything else. He will have to struggle as a Jew, and you ought to develop in him all the energy he will need for that struggle. Do not deprive him of that advantage."[5] What Freud is describing in this letter is not merely "compensation." It is "overcompensation" in the sense of Alfred Adler's theories with which Freud was wrestling in 1909.

The role played by race and culture in shaping the discussion of obsessive neurosis among clinical psychiatrists is evident. Freud's reading (1914) of the case of the non-Jewish patient who has entered the psychoanalytic literature under the name of "Wolf Man" provides a psychoanalytic parallel. The analysis of the "Wolf Man" is Freud's answer to the debates about obsessive neurosis and dysmorphophobia within the clinical psychiatry of his day. Freud had read his obsessive behavior as associated with "the sacred story [of] . . . the ritual circumcision of Christ and of the Jews in general."[6] Indeed, the sign of circumcision would have been a sign of the "prehistory [in which] it was unquestionably the father who practiced castration as a punishment and who later softened it down into circumcision."[7] Thus the anxiety about circumcision has become by the phylogenetic inheritance of all human beings not just an anxiety experienced by Jews.

When Ruth Mack Brunswick (1897–1946) reanalyzed the "Wolf Man," after the publication of Freud's study, she found that his new "hypochondriacal paranoia" focused on his nose.[8] He "neglected his daily life and work because he was engrossed, to the exclusion of all else, in the state of his nose." She noted that "his life was centered on the little mirror in his pocket, and his fate depended on what it revealed or was about to reveal." The patient's anxiety was keyed to the visibility of his disorder, written as it was on his nose: "At the words 'scars never disappear' a terrible sensation took possession of the patient. . . . There was no way out, no possibility of escape. The words of the dermatologist rang in his ears; scars never disappear. There remained for him only one activity . . . to look constantly in his pocket mirror, attempting to establish the degree of his mutilation." This patient's obsessive concern with what seemed to a contemporary observer as a trivial scar resulting from the removal of a sebaceous cyst on his nose reflects the anxiety of the Jewish child as to his potential castration.

The "Wolf Man" is read as a case of castration anxiety and thus as analogous to the case of "Little Hans." Freud turned the "Wolf Man" into a "Jew" through relating his inner anxieties about castration to the Western culture of circumcision. The publication of the case study, which marked him as an exemplary patient (and which later provided him with a livelihood) presented this reading in the public sphere. Any mark on the nose made such an interpretation seem viable to the patient. Here the relationship between the psyche and external body reflected the psychoanalytic dimension. It is the psyche that made the body "unhappy."

The pattern of argument in both of these cases moves from the marked, external body, altered in some form or another, to the psyche, which finds itself made unhappy by the social meaning attributed to the body. The circumcision of the Jewish child becomes an act that reenforces the inherent anxiety about losing one's penis (according to Freud); the response of the "Wolf Man" to his altered nose seems to be rooted in the meaning that the nose has as a sign of disease and difference in Russian culture (as in "The Nose" [1836] by Nikolai Gogol [1809–1852]) as well as in the racial culture of turn-of-the-century Vienna. How does one make someone unhappy? By making it impossible for him to pass (through circumcision) or by branding him with a sign, the scarred nose, which seems to signify that he has become visible (as a member of a too visible cohort). The meaning of the body read now as a site for unhappiness (anxiety) is linked to the racialization of specific sites on the body.

But the Jew's internalization of society's image of the Jew's body leads in specific organs to psychic damage according Freud and Wittels. One does want to become "like the father," according to Freud's reading of Wittels's aesthetic surgery patient's case, but it is the father's nose and penis that define the father as the source of anxiety. It was neither Freud nor Wittels who supplied the basic model for modern aesthetic surgery to understand the psychological efficacy of their project. Freud had overtly abandoned a somatic model with his dismissal of the trauma theory as the origin for hysteria. This came as a result of Fliess's botched "nose job" on Freud and Freud's patient. The physical body in this revised model could only provide minor reenforcement to existing psychological anxieties, such as the fantasy about castration. Thus psychoanalysis provided an answer other than those of aesthetic surgery and clinical psychiatry to the riddle of treating psychological unhappiness with the body.

6. Alfred Adler's Inferiority Complex

Alfred Adler's (1870–1937) notion of "inferior organs" and then his more generalized notion of the inferiority complex provided a model of the mind for the general psychological discussion within aesthetic surgery during the first half of the twentieth century.[1] Here psychology came to be an ally of aesthetic surgery rather than its competition. The "inferiority complex" by the 1920s came to be the generalized shorthand for that which was "cured" through aesthetic surgery.[2] While present in a rudimentary way in the work of some late-nineteenth-century clinical psychiatrists such as Pierre Janet, the notion of "inferiority" was developed by Adler well before his break with Freud in the fall of 1911. As we have already seen, Adler's views certainly impacted Freud's therapeutic proposal to the father of "Little Hans."

Adler's original understanding of organ inferiority was based on the notion that when there was a biological weakness in an organ or organ system, the weakness either seemed to strengthen the organism by offering "compensation" or so weakening the organism that it became ill and in need of medical intervention.[3] A weak organ was always the source of potential health. For Adler, the compensation of the weak organ does not occur in the organ itself but in the equivalent area of the brain responsible for the functioning of the organ. This argument was very much in line with the discussions of brain localization that were taking place before and during World War I. Organ inferiority can be compensated for by the higher functions of the brain and is thus the basis for the constitution of the health ("happiness") of the psyche. In addition the manipulation or repair of an "organ" could indeed repair the psyche or at least allow the body to reconstitute the psyche in a more efficient (and "happier") way.

Adler's idea of "organ inferiority" is clearly shaped by two competing ideas of the time. The first is Cesare Lombroso's idea that genius and madness were linked through the presence in both of inherited psychopathology.[4] "Genius" was merely a positive presentation of an underlying pathology that would inevitably appear in either the genius or his family as insanity. "Genius" was merely a form of overcompensation for inherited psychopathology. The second notion to shape Adler's view was the diagnosis of "moral inferiority" that clinical psychiatrists, such as Emil Kraepelin, introduced to define the moral decay of individuals with hereditary syphilis.[5] The transmission of syphilis to children by infected adults resulted in children unmistakably marked as criminals by their psychology and physiognomy. The very term "inferiority" (Minderwertigkeit) carries with it this moral quality. The notion of "inferiority" was part of the baggage of Darwinian biology as imported into Germany; the physicians adapted it and applied it in a clinical setting. As we saw, Kraepelin stressed that Jews (in Germany and England) and blacks (in the United States) were marked by specific racial physiognomies as well as perceived moral and mental weakness.

Adler's approach to organ inferiority lent itself to resolving problems such as Julius Cohnheim's paradox about tuberculosis—if, Cohnheim asked, everyone was exposed to (and eventually tested positive for) tuberculosis, why do only certain people develop the disease?[6] "Tuberculosis," Adler writes, "is probably always localized in the inferior organ, an assumption which, if conclusively established would bring many of the doubtful questions relating to heredity, place of entry, and paths of infection, immunity and therapy, nearer to a solution" (2). He comments that the "justification of the problems of heredity in the tuberculosis question is pretty well recognized" (14) and that it is the general weakness of the respiratory system that leads to pulmonary tuberculosis. Such weakness, however, can lead to what Adler labels overcompensation, and the individual can become an actor or singer because of the weakness of the respiratory system. So the individual's psyche focuses on the weak pulmonary mechanism, and because the individual is always aware of it he or she constantly compensates for it.

On November 7, 1906, Freud, in commenting on Adler's thesis of organ inferiority noted that "the neurosis is to be traced back to the disparity between constitutional *Anlage* [disposition] and the demands made on the individual by his culture. The deterioration which is frequently observed in families who move from the country to the city belongs in this category." Freud is referring to what he later called "etiologic supplementary series," in which constitution and experience supplement one another.[7] However, his model is that of the "wandering Jew." Freud saw himself as part of that model having "wandered" from the furthest reaches of the Austro-Hungarian empire to Vienna as a child. Freud tries to move Adler's focus on the constitutional and the (seemingly random) notion of the weakness of organs to the level of superego formation. Freud understands exactly what he is doing. Adler's thesis reenforces the commonly held notion of the congenital weakness of the Jew's body, represented by the Jew's presumed predilection to illness. The somatic model is the most widespread somatic illness, tuberculosis. In the standard European handbook of medical eugenics, written by Baur, Fischer, and Lenz, the authors maintain in the 1920s that tuberculosis is an infectious disease, but one to which certain individuals are predisposed through inheritance. For them, the asthenic constitution, one of Ernst Kretschmer's constitutional types, is the physical mark of this predisposition.[8] One can inherit the predisposition to tuberculosis even though one seems basically healthy.[9]

This European tradition argues that the bacterial explanation misses the constitutional dimension (1: 213). For tuberculosis itself plays a eugenic role, as it "destroys weaker constitutions, specifically the asthenic or hypoplastic constitutions" (2: 22). Here is the "habitus phthisicus," the sick, tubercular body of the Jew, which dominates the discussion. Unsurprisingly, it turns out that entire races can possess the "habitus phthisicus": those groups that have been exposed to the disease for centuries, that have been decimated by it because of their exposure to it, also develop a certain resistance to it, such as the Jews (2: 24). Freud answers this question of particular predisposition by taking the case of circumcision, the ultimate example of group specific behavior, and employing its contemporary translation into "castration" as a way of universalizing the specific. Everyone (read: every male) is afraid of castration, even though the Jews in Western society alone circumcise their male children.

Such organ (read: racial) inferiority can provide the locus for an illness but it can also provide the site of greatest resistance to the illness. Adler sees the question of diagnosing such inferiority as problematic because he subscribes to a physiognomic theory. He sees the external signs (directly perceivable to the eye and sense of touch) as "standing in relationship" to unseen organic inferiority: "These have passed up to the present day under the name of external signs of degeneration, or stigmata" (5). In this sense Adler (like Enrico Morselli) is a follower of Lombroso. The model of organ inferiority reveals itself to be a generalization from Lombroso's mid-nineteenth-century theory of genius: "Decided mental predisposition may be considered over-compensation in an inferior brain. It is this inferior brain which may be inherited. In order to lead to epilepsy there must be further determinations. Criminals, drinkers, imbeciles, inventive people, geniuses, apparently healthy people, who however frequently reveal peripheral or partial forms of inferiority, have to alternate in such families till this stock is destroyed by external circumstances or until an equilibrium is reached which guarantees better vitality" (13). This is a classic representation if covert history of the physical history of the Jews as understood at the turn of the century.

Following the racialized model that defined the "Jew" in terms of infant male circumcision, psychological compensation turns out to be male-gendered for Adler.[10] It is the "exaggerated 'masculine protest'" (ix). It is the male who is particularly at risk for this type of inferiority. It leads to masculine ideals of behavior such as assertiveness, ambition, aggression, and defiance. This is central to Adler's understanding of the impact of organ inferiority, which he evokes in the context of the formation of the "neurotic personality" and the "malformation of the genitals" (9). Such (male) patients understand their inferiority not as a result of organ inferiority (biology) but as a result of their nurturing:

On what does the patient base his feeling of inferiority? Inasmuch as the patient is only able to detect the possibility of relationship between disease predispositions and these organ-inferiorities which force themselves upon his attention he is constantly in the path of conjecture. He will for example not seek the reason for his inferiorities in the disturbances of the

secretions of the glands, but will blame in a general way his
weakness, his stunted growth, his sham education, the small
size or anomalies of his genitals, lack of complete virility, his
effeminacy, the feminine traits of a physical or psychic nature,
his parents, his heredity; at times only lack of love, bad training, deprivation in childhood, etc.[11]

Here Adler is rewriting the case of "Little Hans" removing any
specific reference to racial practice (circumcision) and racial marking, and universalizing the "organ inferiority" to a nonspecific, yet
clearly understood damaged male body, that of the Jewish male.

Adler follows a physiognomic tradition of reading the body as a
means of accessing the psyche which he himself outlines. For the
"somatic inferiority" which he refers to in regard to the "variation,
refinement and decline of an organ" comes to be understood as a
quality not only of the organ but of its surface representation (117).
He writes in a footnote that "the 'value of an organ' likewise becomes a symbol in life's current in which are reflected the past,
present, future as well as the fictive goal in like manner as is the
case with the individual's makeup or with the neurotic symptoms.
The idea of the 'symbolic in a person's appearance' is not a new
one. It has been expressed by Porta, Gall, and Carus" (117 n. 12).
Giambattista della Porta (c. 1535–1615), Franz Josef Gall (1758–
1828), and Carl Gustav Carus are three of the major figures in the
history of Western theories of physiognomy. All read the psyche
in terms of the fixed form of the body. Adler gives this a Darwinian turn when he understands the quality (improvement) of the
organ as "facilitating the preservation of life by more finely graded,
sharply differentiated organs as well as by more refined expedients
of the psyche. Thus it is permitted to us, to regard this sort of more
sensitive peripheral apparatus, its special physiognomy and mimic
as a sign of an imperfection of some organ, as a trace which betrays
a transmitted somatic defect" (130). No complete transformation
is truly possible. Some trace remains, no matter how the psyche
compensates. The body will—must—always betray its race.

Adler's case material is less theoretical in representing the traces
that will betray the body. Thus he presents us with the neurotic
case of a young man who came to him with stammering and depression (130). He was avaricious and had "corresponding sexual

impulses" (130). His stammering was a response to his father's command of language. But his sexuality was determined by his sense of the "smallness of his infantile genitalia as compared with the largeness of the paternal ones," which he experienced as a "lack of masculinity." To this point one can speak of masking of the racial component—all of these qualities are those ascribed to the stereotype of the Jew during this period. But Adler adds the ultimate rationale for this patient's sense of inferiority: "To this may be added that he was of Jewish descent. He had heard certain things about circumcision and harbored the idea that he was also belittled [verkürzt] through the operation. His masculine protest drove him to a degradation of woman, as if he had to give proof to his superiority in this wise . . ." (136). Here Adler provides a very specific idea of what can be and what cannot be altered in the treatment of the patient. As with "Little Hans," the body is so inscribed as to make any type of passing impossible. And the anxiety is projected (as I have argued elsewhere) onto the female as the image of the incomplete, inferior human being. Here one can see how the very notion of inferiority complex grows out of the reversal of the somatic model. The inferior organ (the circumcised body) marks the psyche. Here the psychology of aesthetic surgery can be seen to have its origin in the suppression of notions of race.

Another of Adler's patients suffered from anxiety states, this time migraine and depression (195). He also suffered from cryptorchism, the lack of the development or descending of a testicle: "Up to the fourth year of his life he was dressed in girl's clothes, and during this period he developed the fear that he never would reach the mature state of his father or his older brother, that is, never become a complete man. The marked development of his breasts lent considerable weight to his uncertainty" (198). He saw himself in the "feminine role, along with the nursing which is to be considered a gynecomastia which came up during the dream analysis" (200). Feminization becomes the model for the weak male body, the male body with breasts, but this sign develops more and more complex meanings in other aesthetic surgical settings over time. It is the body of the man that seems to become an analogue of that of the woman—through menstruation, through circumcision, through the presence of breasts.

The shift to an external rather than an internal marker for the origin of "inferiority," while paralleled in Freud's case, clearly takes on different dimensions in Adler's work. Unlike Freud, Adler had converted to Protestantism (in 1904) and needed to see the external world as much more malleable than the internal one. If one could shift the social context for "inferiority" from the actual weakness of the physical organ (read: the circumcised penis) to the perception of the individual, one could manipulate this by shifting the appearance of the individual. This transmutation could be undertaken through conversion or through surgery. Physical change is parallel to religious change in altering the psyche of individuals by allowing them to "pass." The end result in this model is a "happy" person, and such a person is "authentic" within the model of Enlightenment autonomy.

Adler's break with Freud and his conversion also marked his own rethinking of a purely somatic model for the "inferiority complex." In his study of neurotic constitution, written in 1912 under the influence of the philosophy of Hans Vaihinger (1852–1933), he claimed that one lived as if one could attain the idealized goals set for oneself in childhood. You are what you imagine yourself to be, states Vaihinger in more complex and philosophical acceptable language. "Unhappiness" is a problem of your fictive life, rather than your ill organs. Fantasy stands center stage. And the psyche can be changed either through therapy or through the alteration of the body itself. If one is primarily what one imagines oneself to be, individual autonomy enables one to be anything one desires to be. And such an imaginary body can be reshaped by aesthetic surgery without any worry about the "realities" of the body. "Inferior organs" become the "inferiority complex."

Adler sketches out this view in his foreword to *New Faces, New Futures* (1936) by the Chicago aesthetic surgeon Maxwell Maltz (1899–1975). In this introduction Adler, now well entrenched in American psychological social work, emphasizes the question of the acceptance of the individual by the peer group. What matters is neither the weakness of the organ nor the question of the actual, physical nature of the individual but "the manner by which the people around him judge others. As we live in a group and are judged by the group, and as this group objects to any departure from normal appearance, it is clear that a facial deformity can have a very deleterious effect on behavior. Fortunately persons thus afflicted need not be permanently handicapped by such external defects, for they can be minimized or entirely removed by the plastic surgeon."[12] Here Adler evokes a version of his own position that "every person should experience the validity and normality of his organs and of his body as a whole." But, of course, the meaning ascribed to the "organ" has shifted from its *actual* weakened or ill state to the psychological sense of unhappiness associated with the collective's representations of the nature of the "organ." It is not that you are sick, it is only that you believe others about the "ugly" nature of your body!

Thus, according to the self-consciously Jewish aesthetic surgeon Maxwell Maltz, it is the surgeon who enables this individual to pass.[13] He writes in *New Faces, New Futures:* "The surgeon . . . seeks to ease the mind by remolding the . . . features to a conformity with the normal. Once normality is attained, the mind throws off its burden of inferiority, of fear of ridicule and of economic insecurity . . . [, and] behavior responds to normal social contacts, the personality relaxes into naturalness and character is transformed" (303). Maltz's view expands that of Adler—he stresses that "passing" enables the individual to be economically secure and free of ridicule—code words for the construction of undesirable social categories. This volume, like Adler's own work, rests on a series of cases in which the specific cultural reading of the body part is central. Central to Maltz's argument is the freeing of the Jews from the curse of "nostrility" and therefore of mental anguish. He states that only 15 percent of all Jews living have a "Jewish" nose (58). Thus the curse of Jewish mental illness as a result of the nature of the Jew's body, evoked as a "genetic" principle by the clinical psychiatrists and accepted by the psychotherapists as a sign of the internalization of the representation of the Jew in Western society, is eliminated as a problem. Since only 15 percent of Jews have a "Jewish nose," it is not a mark on the psychology of the entire cohort. However, Maltz provides his reader with the case study of a woman, showing that the reduction of the size of a too large nose improves not only the psyche of the patient, but also the quality of her voice. She no longer sounded "different." She had become a "new person" and quickly married (67–69). Maltz's sense of the need to correct such noses is linked to his desire not to label them as the source for the inferiority complex of the Jews. Jewish "madness," so powerfully present in the clinical psychiatry of the day, is no longer a simple reflex of Jewish biology, whether of the biological inheritance of the Jews or the outward sign of that biology, the Jewish nose.

The "inferiority complex" quickly becomes the rationale for the aesthetic surgeon. The American reconstructive surgeon Vilray Papin Blair (1871–1955) commented in 1926 that "anything that attracts notice to a child in an unpleasant way is, as a rule, bad for the child. Only those who have dealt with a great number of such children can appreciate how unhappy they can be and how great a permanent damage may result from an inferiority complex."[14] The result of aesthetic surgery can be "increased attention to personal appearance and dress, an infusion of confidence evident in bearing, and a losing of sensitiveness which sometimes amounts to an inferiority complex," according to George Warren Pierce, the San Francisco surgeon.[15] The real pain is the "mental anguish due to the patient's constant realization of the defect which in turn causes the development of an inferiority complex."[16] Thus the inferiority complex becomes part of the foundational discourse of aesthetic surgery, co-opting psychology into the service of aesthetic surgery.

Part of the adaptation of the idea of inferiority is linked to an older model of health and beauty. The Cornell anatomist Charles R. Stockard published his *The Physical Basis of Personality* in 1931, summarizing the standard view that read into Adler's psychology the assumptions of the aesthetic dichotomy between health/beauty and illness/ugliness. Stockard's views (rooted in his work on the "character" of animals and their appearance) were stated in the language of eugenic "science." He writes concerning the nature of "beauty" and "ugliness":

> Ugliness and beauty are frequently observed in the same individual under different physiological states. Any chronic disease may mar the beauty of the fair. As the Germans express it, *Schönheit bedeutet Gesundheit*, beauty indicates health. . . . If we understand what makes a happy person temporarily melancholy, we may surmise something of the state which induces

permanent melancholia in another individual. Goodness and badness, honesty and dishonesty, in common parlance, may, in certain cases at least, result from differences in functional states.[17]

Temporary melancholia is the state of unhappiness that can be remedied by aesthetic surgery, at least according to the surgeons cited at the beginning of this section. Illness can be the cause of such unhappiness, when it affects how the body appears to the self and others. Alter the cause of illness, and beauty (and goodness) result. Beauty becomes health and the problem of organ weakness is seen as a model for psychopathology in general. Stockard's constitutional arguments avoided questions of race directly, but it is clear that bodies that have an inherited constitutional tendency toward the weakness of one or more organs would also have an inherently unhappy psyche. That he extends "unhappiness" to the sphere of criminality is the basis of seeing aesthetic surgery as a cure for sociopathic personalities. Funny-looking noses the criminal make. But what happens when the body is the site of multiple or total disfigurements? Can one change the psyche when one needs to completely alter the body? What happens when happiness and beauty are seen as interchangeable with health? For the answer to these questions, Adler turned to aesthetic surgery.

Adler's theories were used as the rationale for the reconstitution of beauty and happiness through aesthetic surgery. The adaptation of theories of inferiority as the model for the popularization of aesthetic surgery takes place in the 1920s and 1930s. This was only half the story, however, because as we have seen, the Adlerian notion of organ inferiority could be (and also was) used to provide an argument against the amelioration of the psyche through the correction of the body. Thus the American sociologist William E. Carter stated in 1926 that "all the behavior manifestations of the constitutionally inferior can be paralleled from the clinical records of children who are organically normal. An 'unfair deal,' for example (real or imaginary, familial, social or racial), is a frequent source of behavior difficulties."[18] "Must the individual actually have an inferiority as the basis for an inferiority complex? Or is it only the individual who has no actual inferiority who can suffer from the inferiority complex?" asked the psychiatrist Lawson Lowry in seeming confusion, before answering that social conditions were the more dominant in shaping the psyche.[19]

Following the watershed that marked the introduction and general acceptance of the idea of a psychology of aesthetic surgery as rooted in the unconscious, Walter de la Mare (1873–1956), in his 1925 ironic fantasy of Sam Such, the little boy who came to believe that his nose was wax, presents the source of the patient's unhappiness as a problem of parents and children. His parents' belief that their son had a wax nose turned their Sam Such into a recluse and a social misfit—one could not go out in public with a wax nose.[20] (How much of an echo the 1920s scandals about Robert Gersuny's use of paraffin in the reconstruction of the syphilitic nose had on this image one can only imagine. The paraffin eventually distorted the entire face or even killed the patient.[21]) This argument was a psychological one (which is not surprising because it was developed after the introduction of the definition of the "unhappiness" of the patient as an "inferiority complex"). It was not the real nose but the understanding and belief in the meaning associated with the nose that made the child "ill." The answer is not psychotherapy, but rather "reality testing," to use another concept from psychiatry. For it was a physician who inadvertently "cured" his patient by placing him before a roaring fire, which did not melt his "wax" nose. Here the "nose" is quite real but it is the belief about the nose that makes it the source of unhappiness. The image of the "false nose" in the history of the syphilitic nose evoked a deep-seated anxiety about disease and its implication. Here this anxiety is shown to be symbolic and "purely" psychological. As with all cases of the psychoanalytic model, it is the psychological state of the characters that must be the center of attention.

7. Paul Schilder's Social Body

Adler's work in the United States, while completed after the war, had its roots in a prewar Central European understanding of the complex meanings associated with the body. The horrors of World War I and the function of the shattered face in the popular understanding of that event came to refashion the meanings associated with aesthetic surgery after 1919. In the psychological literature the role and meaning of aesthetic surgery as a means of actually "operating on the soul" came to be more and more important after the war.

The American surgeon Adalbert Bettman began to rethink the assumptions of the reconstructive surgeons who performed surgery to heal the wounds suffered during the war. For surgeons who had served in circumstances of war, it was evident that the reconstitution of function could mitigate most psychological trauma in the normal patient. In terms of war, that meant returning soldiers "fit to fight" to the front. The reconstitution of such a level of functioning was seen as a psychological "cure." Similar cures of "shell shock" were undertaken by the psychiatrists to return the soldier to the front. "Cure" was not a return to the "normality" of the civilian, but to that of the soldier.

In implied contrast to the cases of facial war wounds and their seemingly concomitant psychological damage and cure, Bettman sees the preoccupation of one of his patients, an attorney, with a saddle nose to be out of proportion to the physical defect. As a surgeon, Bettman employs the model of the inferiority complex to give meaning to the symptom, rather than a diagnosis of dysmorphophobia:

An attorney had a slight saddle nose. He imagined that juries watched his nose and his efficiency was impaired. His request for relief was stated in these words: "I want you to take my nose out of my mind." The insertion of a piece of rib carti-lage into the bridge removed the deformity, and eight months later he had forgotten his nose. [There is something remotely Gogol-like in that sentence.]

His neurosis undoubtedly resulted from the knowledge that many saddle noses are due to syphilis, and he imagined that everyone else knew this and silently accused him of having this disease. To him his nose became the symbol of syphilis, and he wished a nose which would belie syphilis and cover up his syphilis-complex.[1]

Bettman believed that with the correction of the attorney's defor-mity his inferiority complex was removed. Bettman drew on the symbolic and social significance of the body as the point of origin for "neurosis." The external world that the patient believed defined the normal saw him as different, as diseased. For Bettman, the cor-rection of this neurosis would follow the elimination of the public sign of the patient's illness, his saddle nose. With this act he could "pass" as healthy. Such an approach demanded an emphasis on the social function of the body and rejected any assumption of the sym-bolic or imaginary role of the body as constituted by the psyche.

Reconstructive surgeons turned to aesthetic surgery after World War I and spread the gospel of the repair of the psyche through the correction of the body. The innovative New Zealand reconstruc-tive surgeon Harold Delf Gillies, addressing an American audience in 1934, appealed to his audience:

I ask my surgical colleagues to reconsider their attitude toward aesthetic, reconstructive surgery. . . . The size of the hump of the nose bears little relation to the misery of the patient and to the wisdom of advising its removal. The individual again has to be judged on his merits. Quite frequently some well-known actor or actress takes to the films and discovers some photographic blemish in the line of the nose which is indistin-guishable by the usual camera tricks. The patient's livelihood would depend on a successful removal and even when, as I have known, patients would not dream of having the operation if it were not for their work, I think it would still be justifiable. Even in ordinary life a nasal defect may produce such an inferiority complex as genuinely to hinder the patient's happiness and progress. There is a well-known class, however, which has a nasal complex not relieved by operation, however successful, and such patients are to be avoided. But the differential diagnosis between the genuine and the false is one of considerable difficulty. The help of the psychologist is of great value when there is any doubt.[2]

Gillies's assumption that the social and psychological "happiness" of the patient is the goal and that the psychologist is the natural partner of the aesthetic surgeon shows the unmistakable impact of Adler on the reconstructive surgeon's conception of his task. But it is also clear that he has listened to the clinical psychiatrists, who claim to be able to distinguish between an inferiority complex and an obsessive neurosis. Elsewhere, Gillies writes simply of the "plastic surgery of the psyche."[3] The Adlerian model begins to be expanded from the reconstructive surgery of a damaged "organ" to that of aesthetic surgery.

The social dimension came to be highlighted as can be seen in the provisional constitution of the Society for Plastic and Reconstructive Surgery, adopted in October 1932. One of the basic premises was to "stress the great social, economic, and psychological importance of this surgical specialty."[4] These American views echo the views of aesthetic surgeons in Europe, such as Gillies. Operating on the body is indeed operating on the mind. However, the social and economic dimensions demanded more complex theories than were offered by Adler.

Adler, it may be remembered, posed the question as to whether organs could actually be improved by medical intervention or whether the desire to change the unchangeable would necessarily result in overcompensation. Paul Schilder (1886–1940), one of Freud's former colleagues at the University of Vienna, presented a complex answer to Adler's dilemma. Schilder went to New York University, where in 1935 he revised and expanded his views of body imagery in his book *The Image and Appearance of the Human*

Body, which details the complex interaction between the realities of the body, the perception of the self, and the representation of the self within culture. Schilder's work transcended the popular reception of the Adlerian notion of the inferiority complex by stressing the complex interaction among multiple factors that go into shaping our awareness of our bodies. Never before or since has there been as complex a presentation of the case for the dominance of psychotherapy over aesthetic surgery.[5]

Paul Schilder divides his account of "the picture of our own body which we form in our mind" (11) into three interrelated "bodies"— a physiological body, a psychoanalytic body, and a social body. The first segment of the work focuses on the questions of the physical nature of the body, of body tone and posture as the universal experience of the body. His point of departure is the pathological body. He examines patients with severe neurological disorders that impact their self-perception. His work is heavily indebted to that of the neurologist Kurt Goldstein (1878–1965), who examined soldiers severely wounded during World War I. (One can add that the more recent work of the neurologist Oliver Sacks [1933–] builds on this type of neurological case study as pioneered by Goldstein and Alexander Romanovich Luria [1902–1977].) In patients with devastating wounds to the brain, he was able to work out not only a localization of function, but also of altered relationship to the intact body. Goldstein's work was augmented by work on "phantom limbs" following World War I, where the psychic existence of amputated limbs provided some sense of the body image, that internalized sense of the body that all of us evolve as part of normal development.

Schilder's interest in documenting the "normal" sense of the self led him to experiment with the phenomenon of autoscopy or self-representation. He asked subjects "to imagine themselves with closed eyes standing or sitting in front of themselves" (84) and provide him with a verbal account of what they saw. Their account of their own bodies is cast in aesthetic terms. They imagine themselves "more like a picture, sometimes smaller" (84). What Schilder is aware of is that this exercise provides a "spiritual, inner eye" into the subjects' imaginary construction of their body. It can look inside as well as outside of the body. For Schilder such a mental activity sketches the physiological body, which is never separate from the other two dimensions that he understands as making up the total human sense of self.

The second body is the "libidinous" or psychoanalytic body. This body consists of the drives and their manifestations within the body. Following Freud, Schilder sees the totality of the narcissistic libido as defining this body. It is a body that focuses initially only within itself (119). There is no external world. For Schilder the ambiguity that this internal life gives to the physical body is best understood in our experience of the surface of the body, of the skin. Here Schilder unknowingly begins to construct his libidinous body as a social body, which is, of course, a basic aspect of his own system.[6] He does so by drawing on the social stereotypes of race that dominated the discourse of the body in his time. Schilder does not see these three bodies as in any way separable. They constitute one single, ever changing body image.

In imaging the skin as a part of the libidinous body, Schilder begins to describe the social body. For Schilder we "are unable to obtain a clear conception of the color and texture of the skin" (144). We may even look "into the mirror and still not be sure what we look like." However, and this is central to any understanding of Schilder's concept of the body, there is an exception for him: "It is remarkable that I do not experience the same uncertainty about the skin of colored people." His explanation is that the "racial difference probably diminishes the erotic interest" (144). This view is a commonplace of the psychological literature of the age, having its most evident statement in the work of Havelock Ellis who believed that "racial difference" vitiated erotic interest. Yet it is clear that the Jews, and Schilder was Jewish, were "seen" as possessing precisely the "skin" that was marked as different, both in terms of its skin color and its perceived marks of disease and infection. What Schilder "sees" on his own body is the universal, always changing libidinous, erotic body; the body of the Other is essentially unerotic and therefore unchanging. Schilder cannot read on his own Jewish body the marks of race that in Vienna and in New York his medical colleagues most easily were able to read as signs of the Jew's body.

Schilder's case material seems to provide more than a subtle hint about the ambiguity of the observer's body. The long case study that Schilder provides for this section is that of Francis E., from a "cultivated and emancipated Jewish family," who learns from his Catholic governess at the age of five to hate Jews because they allegedly crucified Christ (150). His hostility to his violent and aggressive parents is manifested in mutual masturbation with his older brother during which they shouted: "Kill the Jews" (151). Jews were "repulsive to him," and after college he converted to Catholicism. No aesthetic surgery is mentioned in this case to alter the body, but the anxiety about pain and its implication for the body results in social transformation, in conversion.

In Schilder's reading, the vocabulary of race provides only symbolic value for this case, which he uses to represent the sadism and masochism of libidinal investment. Thus his account parallels Freud's case of the psychotic Dr. Schreber who, according to Eric Santner, so closely identified with the Jews that he felt himself becoming one.[7] Schilder's patient translates the physical pain of the father's childhood beatings and enemas, using Adler's model (185), into specific forms of psychic pain. All organic change, according to Schilder, is converted into changes in the body image (183). This interrelationship between the body and the psyche is absolute, with changes affecting both depending on the power of the psychological desire.

The final body for Schilder is the social body, which we have already seen shaping his notion of the internal, libidinous life. When he imagines the impact of the social context on the body image, he stresses the function of the social image of the body in deforming the individual's body image in the light of external fantasies about the body. For him "body images are never isolated. They are always encircled by the body images of others" (240). These images "are on principle social" (240). He uses the work of social scientists of the 1920s who examined the construction of cohorts and finds that this construction is closely linked to the construction of the body image. Central to this construction of the social body is "imitation" (245). The members of the cohort imitate the "conviction, feelings, and actions" of the older members of the cohort. The collective body thus forms the individual body through the formation of the superego. This "collective" not only defines the body image for those within the group but can be understood as determining the "out group's" image of its own collective body, too.

The categories in which Schilder expresses the nature of his bodies are those of beauty and ugliness: "Beauty can be a promise of complete satisfaction and can lead up to this satisfaction. Our own beauty or ugliness will not only figure in the image we get about ourselves, but will also figure in the image others build up about us and which will be taken back again into ourselves. . . . Beauty and ugliness are certainly not phenomena in the single individual, but are social phenomena of the utmost importance" (267). The basis for our sense of our own body image lies in the standards of beauty of the cohort. Schilder's case study for this section is telling.

In this final section of his study, Schilder recounted the case of A. M., a twenty-nine-year-old male, whose complaint was that he was "too ugly and that no girl who was in any way attractive ever fell in love with him." His "nose was particularly offensive to him since it was in his opinion too Jewish" (258). He associated this with "his father's family because of their very Semitic appearance and specific Jewish qualities." Appearance became associated for Schilder's patient with a specific negative disposition and this in turn with his own ugliness and his sexual rejection by a young woman. Jewishness sensed on the body becomes converted into ugliness of the spirit. As a result he undertook to have his nose re-shaped by an aesthetic surgeon.

Schilder's analysis with A. M. revealed that the "nose"—following Freud's earlier view—represented the family of his father whose "Semitic" features and resultant character marked him in his fantasy. In the course of his analysis, Schilder tied the anxiety about the father within to the analysand's own sense of the inferiority of his own body. Schilder evokes the classic model of castration anxiety, noting that the patient "when he was young saw his father's sex organ which seemed too big to him. A few years later the thought came to him that his own organ was too small." Thus the analysand came to see "beauty only in the body of others and [he] missed it in his own body." His drive for an aesthetic in himself was limited by the sense of the inferiority of his body—of the presence in his internalized sense of himself of the body of the father, and the symbol of the father's body was the nose.

But all of these readings of the body are to be understood in the social context of the patient's sense of his or her own body. Beauty and ugliness, as social phenomena, writes Schilder, "regulate the sex activities in human relations, and not only in the manifest heterosexual activities, but also the homosexual ones which are so important for the social structure. In the case of our patient, the admiration for his friends who were, in his opinion, better endowed than himself, plays an enormous part. Our own body image and the body image of others, their beauty and ugliness, thus become the basis for our sexual and social activities. We like to believe that our standards of beauty are absolute" (268). Schilder sees the patient only after his rhinoplasty. The patient "quoted others who said that before his operation his face was more characteristic [read: Jewish] than it was now, but seemed on the whole rather contented with the result." The operation itself is the social act that enabled the patient to come to terms with the immutability of his Jewish body. No matter what is done, the body will always reveal itself to be that of a Jew. This crushing realization drives the patient beyond medicine for therapy. A. M. eventually breaks with his racial-religious identity and converts to Catholicism, the ultimate form of passing in Catholic Vienna. Aesthetic surgery did not "cure" the patient of his "Jewishness," it only masked it. Baptism became the answer for A. M. But as we have seen in the case of Fritz Wittels's patients, conversion itself was a fruitless attempt to alter the immutable signs of race and was understood as a sign of psychopathology. There was no escaping from the self-awareness of one's Jewish identity in the Vienna of Sigmund Freud.

The therapy outlined by the aesthetic surgeons—to have the rhinoplasty serve as a part of the therapy—seems not to work here; nor can we reduce this patient to the desire to distance himself from his father's nose and identity; nor is it an inferiority complex, which results from a sense of the social stigma associated with being seen as different. A. M.'s resolution is one that we have seen elsewhere in Schilder, a desired social transformation through the act of conversion. Rhinoplasty becomes one of the means for attempted transformation—but, we can ask, is such a belief in transformation still meaningful or is it another sign of the paranoid disruption of the relationship with reality? Here Schilder locates aesthetic surgery, as part of the medical-social reality that alters the body image but cannot truly change the psyche. There is a limitation on such somatopsychic therapy. Altering the "ill" organ works in this system only when the notion of a physical weakness or illness is present. The symbolic illness represented by the Jewish nose and the internalization of its meaning in Vienna cannot be "cured" through surgery. The result is a continuation of the neurosis, represented by the act of conversion. Schilder gives the reader two major case studies of males with anxiety about their (read: his) Jewish appearance and identity. Both end in conversion and are thus "failures" since the transformation is sought in the society rather than in the self. Aesthetic surgery cannot cure the mind; only psychotherapy can cure the distorted body image and make one come to terms with the essential self.

8. Karl Menninger's Polysurgery

Orthodox psychoanalytic literature of the 1930s and 1940s continued to read into the desire for aesthetic surgery the unconscious, symbolic desires and fear of castration. This desire was clearly marked by Freud and the early psychoanalytic commentators as "Jewish," following the pattern in the case of "Little Hans." Following Freud's lead in the discussion of the Wittels's case, psychoanalysts of the second and third generations sought out the "hard cases," those that did not show psychic improvement through the initial procedures as their counterfactuals to the psychological theories of the aesthetic surgeons.[1] Yet the impact of aesthetic surgery on psychoanalysis was itself becoming evident.

There was an increased interest in the psychoanalytic literature of this period in what Karl A. Menninger (1893–1990) in 1934 called "polysurgical addiction," those patients, including aesthetic surgical patients, who seemed to have a compulsive need for surgical interventions.[2] For the aesthetic surgeons even in 1996 the question of patients' desiring multiple procedures is vital, since in that year 21 percent of the 1,937,877 patients of the members of the American Society of Plastic and Reconstructive Surgery were "repeat patients." How does one separate those patients who will profit from multiple procedures from those whose search for perfect (in)visibility means they will never be satisfied?

Menninger's paper was the first psychoanalytic attempt to outline the parameters for any discussion of aesthetic surgery in American culture, and he does so in the general context of "polysurgical" addiction. Menninger quite clearly understood the psychological impact, especially on a child, of being brought "into a strange white room, surrounding him with white-garbed strangers, exhibiting queer paraphernalia and glittering knives and at the height of his consternation pressing an ether cone over his face and telling him to breath easily" (173). This scene, more reminiscent of a meeting of the Ku Klux Klan than a place of healing, provided Menninger with a "natural" case study.

Given the Klan's notorious practice of castration, Menninger tells the tale of a twenty-eight-year-old man who had been taken to the hospital at age three because "my father accused me of masturbating" (174). He told a neighbor, "We're going to the doctor to have my punanny cut off." Taken to the hospital, he was circumcised as a therapy/punishment for masturbating. Many years later, suffering from depression, he was asked by his physician whether he masturbated. The result of the question was that he fell into a catatonic state and awoke in a state mental hospital desirous of being castrated. This reenactment of the anxiety of Little Hans enabled Menninger to place "castration anxiety" at the center of the male desire for repetitive surgery. For the patient was able to turn the anxiety about his castration (and circumcision) into a part of his erotic fantasy world. While Menninger's patient did not have any further "surgery," that is, he was not castrated in the hospital, Menninger sees the unwilling reenactment of the anxiety of the initial surgery in terms of the adult's world of erotic fantasy. What had been inflicted upon the patient earlier was now desired by the patient.

In addition to castration anxiety, Menninger postulates three other psychological motivations for repeated surgery. For Menninger, if men undertake surgery to prove that they can be castrated and also are able to turn that anxiety about castration into an "erotic capitalization" then, for him, women undertake surgery to "fulfill an ungratified infantile wish for a child" (183). This transformation of the male anxiety of loss into the female desire for reproduction came about through the association of both with hospitals in an age in which childbirth had moved from the home to the hospital as a sign of the modern. Finally, he noted that the patient undertakes surgery "to avoid facing something else which he fears more" (178). Patients transfer the father and the father's idealized qualities onto the surgeon: "The incisiveness, firmness, strength—one might almost say ruthlessness—of the surgeon, and the general mental and physical superiority common to so many surgeons" (181). The surgeon as father and the patient as child provide a model that is hardly conducive to cure. It rather evokes the world that, according to Freud, produces neurosis and psychosis instead of curing the psyche through intervening in the body.

Menninger's message to the surgeons is clear. He quotes "with astonishment an influential middle-age surgeon" saying, "You can't get things out of people's minds with surgery. You've got to get it out with psychoanalysis" (175). The fixation on the body is the symptom that signals the therapeutic intervention of the psychoanalyst not the surgeon. Given the competition between the aesthetic surgeons and the psychoanalysts for the mind and body of the patient, the admission of a surgeon that psychoanalysis is a more efficient means of therapy than surgery places the analyst in the superior professional position.

Despite Menninger's privileging of psychoanalysis over surgery, he makes a rather important distinction in his paper, of which he himself seemed not to be aware. Menninger placed aesthetic surgery in a special category. This is evoked by his paraphrase of Freud's comment, in *Beyond the Pleasure Principle*, that illness or physical injury can relieve specific forms of mental illness, such as traumatic neurosis, depression or schizophrenia, through binding the libido caused by the unprepared event. This is the basis for contemporary treatments of mental illnesses such as malaria therapy. Menninger himself creates a special category for aesthetic surgery and those who repeatedly undertake it. He begins by exempting from the category of polysurgery "the frequent operations necessary in certain bone diseases and plastic surgery where the greater the skill of the surgeon, perhaps, the more attenuated and gradual the technique" (176 n). Such "reconstructive" procedures demand multiple interventions and are permitted. But reconstructive procedures are seen as different in nature from aesthetic surgery, as his contemporaries would have understood.

To undertake his study of "polysurgery," Menninger actually visited an aesthetic surgeon, H. L. Updegraff in Hollywood, California, and reported on two of his patients. The first is a forty-year-old schoolteacher who requests an operation to reduce "a slight enlargement" of her labia, complaining of somatic disorders and anxiety about developing cancer. Menninger uncovered that she was about to marry a childhood sweetheart who had reappeared after a fifteen-year absence and with whom she was on "terms of exhibitionist intimacy." She wished to have her labia reduced because she believed that her masturbation had led to their enlargement and that she would be revealed to her lover as a chronic masturbator. Menninger reports that "a minor removal of the excess tissue gave her complete relief, both mentally and physically" (187). A single procedure produces a happy patient.

Updegraff's second patient was a man, "a Jewish merchant," who presented with a request to have his nose reconstructed because he claimed that a childhood injury gave him a "pugilistic appearance" (188). There is a desire here to pass that underlies the anxiety about looking like a boxer. Ernest Hemingway's Robert Cohn in *The Sun Also Rises* (1926) came "out of Princeton with painful self-consciousness and the flattened nose" he got boxing to prove that even a Jew could do sports.[3] The "real" problem with the appearance of his nose has little to do with looking as if he did sports.

Menninger saw the "merchant" only after the procedure that had relieved him of "feelings of anxiety and 'isolation.'" This is, once again, an example of someone who had had a single procedure and supposedly became a happy patient. The patient told Menninger that before the procedure he had a dream in which the operation left his "nose larger and uglier so that he was 'hideously deformed.'" The guilt that Menninger sees in this dream seems to belie the success of the procedure in psychological terms. Through "analysis" (evidently a single session), Menninger revealed that the patient had stopped an affair with a "Jewish girl" and had begun one with a "Gentile girl" prior to the rhinoplasty. This had caused him "great depression and it was in this depression that he consulted the surgeon in regard to an operation." His "strong conflict on the Jew-Gentile question" led to a feeling of guilt as he saw his relationship with the non-Jewish woman as "an effort on his part to deny or relinquish his Jewishness" (188). Here the question of reading the success of the operation ceases. Menninger does not explore why the procedure, which left the merchant looking "better," also resolved his conflict about his Jewish identity. As with the first patient, the successful intervention is examined only in terms of its initial, hidden motivation, not the radical success of its cure.

Neither case is an example of "polysurgical addiction." When

Menninger does explain polysurgical addiction he does so against the popular image of aesthetic surgery in the 1930s, an image of individuals addicted to such surgery for reasons of vanity. Robert Weir's anomalous case of the 1890s, which we discussed in the opening chapter of this section, had come to be the model for the "unhappy" aesthetic surgical patient, the one who was unhappy with the results of surgery because of a psychological predisposition (dysmorphophobia). The early procedures, according to the surgeons, seem to be very successful in reducing the unhappiness of most patients. For Menninger, however, his "Hollywood" cases of aesthetic surgery almost serve as counterfactuals in his account of polysurgical addiction. They seem to be patients who have had single procedures that "cured" them of the psychological unhappiness.

Menninger's approach is an attempted mediation between aesthetic surgery and psychoanalysis. Aesthetic surgery is the one place in Menninger's paper where surgery seems not only appropriate as a means of somatopsychic therapy but actually has immediate and positive psychological results. Menninger's "happy" patients thus violate the "middle-aged surgeon's" dogma about psychoanalysis as the one place to cure the psyche. Rather, in the United States in the 1930s, the competition between aesthetic surgery and psychoanalysis could also be resolved into cooperation. Both approaches were understood as modern, as European, as curative. His two cases, like Stekel's cases of obsessive neurosis, provide two gender-specific readings of the positive effect of aesthetic surgery. Each is in its own way an answer to Menninger's initial rewriting of the case of Little Hans. Here the "Woman Question" and the "Jewish Question" are resolved through the happiness attendant on aesthetic surgery.

If the overall claim was that surgery did not cure the psyche, only psychotherapy did, how do therapists deal with surgery? Helene Deutsch (1884–1982) claimed to see in her own patients the negative result of surgical interventions.[4] She comments that "the percentage of analytic patients who have had operations before they come to analysis is extraordinarily high" (105). Much of her analysis is concerned with relieving the anxiety created by the earlier surgery. Surgery did not make the patient happy, according to such views; rather, it exacerbated the impossibility of happiness through the patient's experience of trauma. None of this surgery, as she tabulates it, is aesthetic surgery. Hers is the opposite model to Freud's original idea of psychoanalysis prior to 1895. There trauma led to physical symptoms, which were alleviated by the "talking cure." The idea of a fantasy that is shaped by the experience of trauma, which is where Freud eventually lands in his thinking, seems to have been modified to a degree.

Deutsch agrees with Menninger's notion of castration anxiety's being at the core of male anxiety about surgery. She also claims that the fantasy may differ from individual to individual and that men might experience surgery in different ways. Passive men experience surgery as "a delivery, just as it is in women" (114). The experience of surgery is determined by the existing "character" of the patient rather than being shaped by it. The trauma of surgery seems only to awaken existing psychic patterns. Here psychoanalysis supervenes and can be the ultimate treatment.

Should the psychoanalyst, therefore, become the collaborator of the surgeon? Can psychotherapy provide interventions that are needed before as well as after surgery? The end result of Deutsch's deliberations is to forfeit any role as the collaborator of the surgeon: "Often we psychiatrists are absolutely helpless when we are approached for advice. . . . In the patient I discussed in detail the psychiatrist understood all the psychic determinants, he could not decide to give a contra-indication for the surgical procedure and so perhaps endanger the patient's life." But what of procedures that do not endanger the patient's life? What about aesthetic surgery? Such elective procedures seem not to follow the pattern of "real" surgery.

The example that closes Deutsch's argument parallels that of Menninger's opening case study: "If surgeons only knew how much damage is done, for example, by a circumcision performed as a hygienic measure during the early years of childhood, they would feel like so many Herods. Modern pediatricians are beginning to take the state of infantile anxiety into account before deciding on any operation which is not absolutely necessary" (115). Is this the one case of crypto-aesthetic surgery in her argument? Here is Deutsch's answer to the question of aesthetic surgery, cast in the form of circumcision for hygiene (rather than as ritual). For her, if one can understand the psychological dimension, then the totality of the procedure can be grasped. Her language is biblical and her reference is to the Massacre of the Innocents. Her opposition seems to be rooted in the anxiety about disguise felt by German Jews who circumcised their children ritually.[5] All become one with the anxiety about passing and seeing the body as different.

Erich Lindemann (1900–1974) came to understand that any violation of the body engenders exacerbated neurosis even in the normal patient.[6] Lindemann's forty female patients had major abdominal, not aesthetic surgery. What he found was that the patients who were less stable prior to their initial surgery suffered from the greatest psychological trauma following surgery. He concluded: "For these findings one might anticipate that a woman who is independent and controlling, who hates the aging process (which is out of her control), who hopes the operation will slow it down, and who has evidence of depressive symptoms preoperatively will have an intensification of her depressive symptoms in the immediate postoperative period" (132). According to contemporary commentators, this would be the case in some women having face-lifts, yet Lindemann avoids this conclusion. The model of surgery that Lindemann presents is one that is clearly delimited: "Surgical operations present a well-defined trauma consisting of anesthesia, mechanical injury, possible removal of certain organs, and alteration of psychological function set up by the injury" (132). Aesthetic surgery is, by this definition, not really "surgery."

If we apply the Talcott Parsons (1902–1979) standard sociological definition of the "patient role," aesthetic surgical patients are not really patients[7] (which is one of the reasons that most government systems and third-party insurers do not cover aesthetic surgery). There is little "gain from illness" in such patients. Indeed, many of them even refuse to acknowledge having had a procedure and thus forfeit the sympathy one gains from being ill. For such patients the prognosis in terms of morbidity and mortality is almost ideal; people rarely are incapacitated or die from such procedures. Patients have their procedures under local anesthesia. There is little anticipated pain, and, foremost, it is the patient, not the physician, who judges the success of the procedure.

Why then do other surgical patients refuse to become "happy" through surgical intervention? Phyllis Greenacre (1894–1989) stressed that the surgical intervention exacerbated the original neurosis, encapsulating it and making the addiction to future surgery possible.[8] By analogy, contemporary thinkers see this as a problem of the definition of the unsuccessful psychological outcome of aesthetic surgery even into the present. In a detailed study by Knorr, Edgerton, and Hoopes at the Johns Hopkins University's Division of Plastic Surgery and Psychiatric Liaison Service, the qualities of the "bad" patient are enumerated in detail.[9] Based on a questionnaire completed by 325 surgeons, this empirical study created an exemplary "bad" or "unhappy" potential patient. The patient was given eleven qualities and was then presented to the surgeons for their comments. The patient profile was of a male, unmarried, twenty to thirty-five years old, with low self-esteem, grandiose ambitions, hyposexual, with no long-term relationships, extremely obsessive, yet passive in dealing with the surgeon, aggressive when not accommodated, anxious, vague about the goals of surgery, dissatisfied following initial postoperative enthusiasm. The problem presented was seen as too minimal. Such patients were understood by only half (55 percent) of the surgeons as counterindicated for surgery. Most saw such patients as psychiatric patients, rather than surgical patients. The result of the paper is the strong advocacy of a collaboration between the surgeon and the psychiatrist for the identification and treatment of such patients.

The ambivalence of the relationship between psychiatrist or psychoanalyst and surgeon came to permeate the technical, surgical literature on aesthetic surgery. Even renowned surgeons such as Vilray Papin Blair (1871–1955) and James Barrett Brown, like the psychoanalysts, came to question the underlying motivation of some of their patients.[10] Freud's mistrust of his neurotics comes to be their model for the mistrust of the polysurgical aesthetic patient by the surgeon. Evoking a basic physiognomic "truth" at the opening of their extensive paper on "nasal abnormalities," they link the social, psychological, and economic status of their patients:

On every countenance is the imprint of the soul, its aims, and its encounters, so that "he that runs may read." At best, however, the reading is not always easy, and, if the page be torn, burnt, or poorly made, the soul might feel that she were unfairly treated, and even desire a change. Should remunerative employment or a change in social status be desired, this change may become a necessity. (797)

While concentrating on patients undergoing reconstructive as well as aesthetic surgery, they also observed that "a patient's inability to state accurately and succinctly the thing that displeases him . . . should excite suspicion that the accused nose might not be the real fault" (797). The act of narration is one of the marks of a healthy psyche. And the nose "is the most conspicuous feature of the face, and any exaggeration, loss, or deformity renders it not only a target for undesired attention, but is not inapt to produce deprecatory or disquieting self-consciousness." These "unhappy" patients may not be able to be cured through aesthetic surgery.

Blair and Brown measure the psychological success of the intervention based on the extreme nature of the fault being corrected: "The more pronounced the deformity of loss, the more apt is a reasonably good result likely to be acceptable" (797). Thus the slighter the defect, the less "happiness" can result and the more evident it is that the patient's problem is not "correctable" through aesthetic surgery. It is better for surgeon and patient "that the desired correction not be attempted." Here the surgeons' perception of the patient's physiognomy becomes a central factor in predicting the positive or negative outcome of the surgery. The smaller the problem (i.e., the more aesthetic the surgery), the smaller the likelihood of a positive outcome. But the relatively smaller success of aesthetic surgery than reconstructive surgery is defined in terms of the state of the art of surgery and the skill of the surgeon:

In rebuilding or in changing a nose, one is dealing with material facts related to anatomy and physiology, and with fundamental rules that have been formulated in regard to the proper ensemble of the facial elements, but, in passing upon the advisability of the attempt, one must also take cognizance of the patient's mental attitude. If that has become a bit warped, it can in the end defeat the main objective, namely, pleasing the patient, regardless of the fact that the newly made nose might be surgically and artistically as near perfection as the available material and our skill permit. (797)

The limitations of procedure and taste on the part of the surgeon may be something to which the patient responds. With a massive deformation, all correction is understood for the better; for aesthetic patients, the possibility of not fulfilling their expectation remains a problem of their psychological response to the always limited ability of the surgeon. And one can imagine, as in the case of Paul Schilder, that the norm is the appearance of the investigator. The more you look like me and want to change, the more likely you are psychopathic.

The psychoanalytic theories dealing with aesthetic surgery provided a label for what it cured: inferiority. The model for the discussion of inferiority arose out of the racialist underpinnings of late-nineteenth-century culture with its competing models of constitutional permanence and social change. If passing was possible, then happiness could be acquired; if it was merely a pipe dream, then no cure of the psyche could be acquired through any intervention that would change the body or its perception. But the observer/physician/surgeon's body served as the unstated norm. Given that many of these individuals belong to visible cohorts (such as Jews) the measurement of the difference of mind and body as signs of health and psychopathology come to be reflexes of the perceived position of the healer in modern society. And we know that the healer must look healthy—otherwise who would come to the healer for succor?

The spread of a psychological theory of aesthetic surgery as the basic rationale for undertaking surgery on a healthy body to correct an unhappy psyche resonates throughout every aspect of Western society. In the setting of those organized religions, such as Judaism, that focus on the role of medicine as part of religious ethics, these questions came to be highly debated, especially as aesthetic surgery became more and more an experience linked to acculturation of Jews (and other ethnic groups) in the United States. The nose job, with its origins in the culture of nineteenth-century racial practice, came to be accepted only so far as the psychological rationale of the inferiority complex was accepted.

Biblical injunctions concerning the face as the place where health and illness, beauty and ugliness are linked provide a rationale for Jewish concerns with aesthetic surgery. In Leviticus 21:18 men with "charum" are forbidden from becoming priests in the Temple. This term appears only in this passage in Leviticus and seems to refers to "something maimed," but cognates from other languages show that this "something maimed" is most likely to be in the face. The Hebrew word "charum" is defined in Bechoroth 7:3 (through Rashi's commentary) as "flat-nosed." The Gemara comments that it means to be snub-nosed. Both the Mishna and the Talmud translate it as "flat-nosed": "The priest that is flat-nosed is unqualified [for Temple service]. What is understood by 'flat-nosed'? It means one that can point both his eyes together." In Bechoroth 7:4 there is another reference to disproportionate noses: "if his nose be too big [compared] with his limbs or too small [in comparison] with his limbs [he is unqualified]." The note to this in the Mishna states that the "nose is so flattened that the nostrils are exposed" and that the "nose between the eyes is so flat that it does not prevent the color running from one eye to the other." In other words, these are signs of physical anomalies that are also represented as unaesthetic. Later commentators observe that this injunction was aimed against those with leprosy who were seen as ritually unclean.[1] The unclean is also the ugly and the unhappy: think of Job's boils.

Traditional Jewish religious views of aesthetic surgery come to focus on the question of the meanings ascribed to transformation of the nose. The Talmud, as in the discussion of "charum" in Leviticus, defines the nose as one of the central organs of the body. Abba Saul notes "that when an embryo is formed it is formed from the center, but with respect to existence all agree that its source is in the nose; for it is written, *All in whose nostrils was the breath of the spirit of life [Genesis 8: 22]*" (Sotah 45b). When it comes to the aesthetic alteration of the body, specifically that of the "Jewish nose," the complex relationship between body and mind is brought to bear on the definition of aesthetic surgery. The alteration of the nose is a serious procedure, but it is permitted if it eliminates "psychological anguish."[2] This acceptance is to be read in the light of the role that such procedures had in creating an acceptable "American" physiognomy for the Jews in both Europe and the United States.

Aesthetic surgery is dealt with within post-Shoah Jewish tradition in such a way as to acknowledge the model developed by the surgeons and the psychologists. Here too there are slight differences in cultural emphasis. One must begin with the observation that traditional Judaism rejects surgical alteration of the body, including the nose, except for reconstructive surgery under the prohibition against "chavalah" (wounding). (Circumcision is a religious and not a medical practice for traditional Jews. Indeed the theological understanding is that had God not commanded its practice, it would not be sanctioned under Jewish law.[3]) Yet what is striking is that halachic traditions would permit the alteration of the shape of the nose for men and for women. Such permission turns on the acceptance of the psychological efficacy of aesthetic surgery.

If we turn to the period during the development of modern aesthetic surgery, we can see that there is already a set of presuppositions within European Jewish religious thought concerning the nature of transformation and its psychological consequences. Parallel to the popular understanding of the mutability of the body, which we discussed earlier in this book, theologians too made this aspect of Jewish thought part of their representation of the "Jew." In 1869, one of the leading Rabbis in Vienna, Adolf Jellinek (1821–1893), wrote of the Jews' ability to mimic the peoples among whom they lived.[4] The mimicry provides the Jew with status, according to Jellinek, and leads to his acceptance within the world of the Jew. The result of such acceptance is the "happiness" of the Jews. Transformation leads to happiness. This is a formula that underlies the discussion of aesthetic surgery, some one hundred years later.

Rabbi Immanuel Jakobovits (1921–), then the rabbi of the Fifth Avenue Synagogue in New York and later the chief rabbi of Great Britain, is an individual greatly concerned with ethical problems of medicine. Trained in medical ethics at the University of London, he came to New York at a point where young Jewish women were receiving rhinoplasties as their usual "sweet sixteen" present. This must have struck him deeply because British society had not yet become part of an international culture of aesthetic surgery. In comparison with American Jewry, British Jewry felt itself to be established in England, and Jews believed they were (in)visible as English men and women walking on the street while still retaining their Jewish culture in their homes (to alter the pre-Shoah German Jewish formulation). Indeed, Jakobovits ended his career as a member of the House of Lords.

In 1962 Jakobovits offered a secular *responsa* that "cosmetic surgery is justified if the defect is such that it 1) prevents a woman from finding a marriage partner, 2) prevents a happy relationship with her husband, or 3) prevents a person from fulfilling a constructive function in society—this applies especially to men who without such improvement could not earn enough to support their families."[5] Yet he also dismisses the psychological argument for an economic one: "I very much doubt if, as a rule, the psychological stress, in merely pathological terms, resulting from the facial malformation to be corrected will outweigh and thus neutralize the health and other risks involved in such an operation. In other words, the chief indication for such surgery, I suspect, is cosmetic pure and simple and not medical" (133–34). He believes that such a procedure would not fall within the interpretation of the Talmudic injunction in Tosafot, Shabbat 50b that states that a state

of mind that prevents a person from mingling with people constitutes "pain" within the halachic definition. The rationale of the
aesthetic surgeons and the psychologists—that the reshaping of the
nose cures the psyche—has become accepted among traditional
Jews who in general would reject any merely cosmetic alteration
of the body.[6]

But Jakobovits also evokes the case of the Renaissance surgeon
Gaspare Tagliacozzi (1545-1599) as an example of the Catholic
Church's intolerance of aesthetic surgery. Tagliacozzi was credited
with having developed in the sixteenth century the first reconstructive rhinoplasty using a connected flap from the arm. His
procedures were lost to European medicine until the end of the
eighteenth century.[7] Jakobovits repeats the myth of the exhuma-
tion of Tagliacozzi's corpse, having been condemned after his death
for his "attempt to improve upon the work of the Almighty" (133).
Since Tagliacozzi too was chastised for his surgical practice, this
is seen as proof that the questions concerning the permissibility
of aesthetic surgery are "a religious problem" and not exclusively a
Jewish one. The theological question is this: "by trying to improve
on God's work and create a human being other than He had created
or intended, do we not attack the scheme of Providence?" (134).
Jakobovits's answer is finally a pragmatic one based on the "amelioration of the lot of many people." This bow to his New York
City constituency is damning with faint praise. Aesthetic surgery
is permissible because it makes individuals happier, but this happiness has already been dismissed at the beginning of his argument.

The American Rabbi J. David Bleich provides a yet more complicated rationale to permit the undertaking of aesthetic surgery.
Bleich teaches medical ethics at the Orthodox Yeshiva University
in New York City. He also begins with the prohibition against
"chavalah" (wounding), noting that there is also a clear prohibition against risking one's life for cosmetic purposes but adds that
some Rabbinic authorities have cited Deuteronomy 22:5. "A man
shall not put on a woman's garment," seeing aesthetic surgery as
gendered.[8] Bleich argues against this threefold rationale to prevent
aesthetic surgery. Citing Tosafot, Shabbat 50b, he also argues that
social isolation constitutes "pain" within the halachic definition.
But unlike Jakobovits, Bleich does not see the simple inability to
marry or to have economic success as sufficient rationale, citing

Tosafot, Baba Kamma 91b, which states that wounding is forbidden when undertaken for pecuniary advantage. Desire for financial gain or finding a marriage partner is not sufficient; yet the "psychological anguish normally attendant upon not being able to find gainful employment or a suitable marriage partner is, for him, a form of 'pain.'" Thus aesthetic surgery is sanctioned only to alleviate psychological anguish; it is not permitted simply for purposes of "beautification." Thus it is permitted for men as well as women (128).

Given Jakobovits's evocation of the supposed history of the Catholic Church's opposition to aesthetic surgery, it is evident that the views of the Roman Catholic Church are today somewhat different from those of Orthodox Judaism. Father Charles G. O'Leary defends aesthetic surgery by evoking the theological "Principle of Totality" in which a part of the body can be sacrificed for the good of the whole.[9] Even if the intent of the procedure is to achieve "physical beauty," the principle holds. You can sacrifice your "too Irish" nose if the end result is a more coherent body, in your own estimation. The moral evaluation of the act must show that the intention must be right; the general health of the patient must not place the patient at risk; and the motives must be proportionate to the means employed. It cannot be sanctioned if the purpose is "mere vanity or fashion" (61). And what is not "mere vanity"? Aesthetic surgery can be sanctioned if it ameliorates "grave psychological effects . . . such as a sense of inferiority." At that point it is not "only permissible but also a necessity."

Here Pope Pius XII can be cited: "If we consider physical beauty in its Christian light and if we respect the conditions set by our moral teachings, then aesthetic surgery is not in contradiction to the will of God, in that it restores the perfection of that greatest work of creation, man."[10] Aesthetic surgery is restorative surgery, restorative to the ideal body, that divine norm against which one measures the weaknesses and faults of real human beings. Such restoration of the body becomes, as far as religious practice permits it, an acknowledgment of its "holistic" reconstitution of the entire person—psyche as well as body. Religious responses take the argument of "happiness" extremely seriously.

10. Prescott Lecky's Self-Consistency

Confronted by religious, clinical, and psychoanalytic rationales for the efficacy or lack of efficacy of aesthetic surgery, the modern aesthetic surgeons, more than any other surgical subspecialists, linked their undertaking to the world of psychology. In no other surgical specialty is psychological testing and evaluation of patients done as commonly as in aesthetic surgery. The extensive use of psychological instruments such as *Minnesota Multiphasic Personality Inventory-2* and personal history questionnaires, such as the *Patient Attitude Scale*, as well as the development of instruments such as the *Expectation for Plastic Surgery Scale*, seems to be unique.[1] Indeed, even the field of aesthetic dentistry has developed a psychological instrument—the *Esthetic Analysis Form*.[2] The intent of such instruments is to identify those who will be helped (made "happy") by various interventions and those who will remain "unhappy" and may then turn to the courts for redress.[3]

This is not only a concern of the present. Charles Conrad Miller (1880–1950), one of the pioneers of facial aesthetic surgery in Chicago before World War I, wrote that "cosmetic surgery appeals to vain people. There are many idle men and women who have nothing to do but study themselves. These people are frequently extremely neurotic and selfish. They will expect marvelous transformations from operations. If the surgeon in this field expects to enjoy peace of mind in his practice he will carefully study character and learn to avoid these psychopaths, for with nothing to do, after an operation which would prove satisfactory to a reasonable person, such patients may work up a degree of discontent which is appalling in its intensity."[4] Miller wrote from personal experience, having been hounded out of the profession of aesthetic surgery by the medical establishment after losing a particularly nasty court case in which the patient remained quite "unhappy."

Such questions of appropriate patient selection are addressed in the much recent literature. Hans-Peter Wengle of the University of Zurich provided an overview of American and European literature on the psychology of aesthetic surgery with special emphasis on controlled studies of the efficacy of aesthetic surgery. He examined "the personal impact of a deformity, differences between subjective and objective assessment of the cosmetic defect, the patient's personality, sex differences in relation to outcome, external versus internal motivation for surgery, severity of cosmetic defect and postoperative psychological results, postoperative patient satisfaction, and psychological complications." Having examined virtually every possible variable presented in the psychological literature, he finally turned to Morselli's and Freud's original question of whether surgery or psychotherapy is the more appropriate treatment modality.[5] In a follow-up study he commented that "none of the criteria [in the existing literature] proves to be statistically significant in regard to the outcome of cosmetic surgery." Wengle, following what has now become more or less common practice for aesthetic surgery, wants to introduce a clearly psychological dimension into the patient selection process. Central to him is a systemic-interactional model of thinking, and he wants to apply it to what he defines as the patient-surgeon-psychiatrist triangle and management of the patient in the screening. At this point the patient who will not be made "happy" through surgical intervention can be identified; those patients for whom passing is truly an impossibility, because they have come, for whatever reason, to believe so very deeply in their own inherent, essential difference, can be weeded out. In addition Wengle sees the surgical procedure as efficacious only when it is literally taken as part of a self-conscious treatment of the psyche. For him aesthetic surgery is truly surgery on the psyche when it literally merges with psychotherapy.

Wengle's views are part of the same call for the psychologist to examine and diagnose the psyche of the aesthetic surgical patient prior to surgery. In a detailed study M. R. Wright and W. K. Wright examined the personality of patients requesting cosmetic rhinoplasty. They began by exposing the patients to a battery of "objective projective" tests and psychological interviews to determine whether "patients seeking cosmetic surgery are not as psychologically disturbed as often as described." This is an attempt to answer the type of studies undertaken in regard to dysmorphophobia in which the intent is to document the psychopathology of the aesthetic surgery patient. The tests weeded out a range of personality disorders, such as "the infantile-narcissistic and the manipulative controlling personalities." The patients operated upon were thus "normal" rather than disturbed according to their scales. When similar scales were applied eighteen months after surgery, no major personality changes were registered but "self-concept was improved." Happiness is an improved self-concept, but only in patients who were essentially "healthy" prior to surgery. They "recommend[ed] a simple interview question method of counseling designed to identify underlying psychological manifestations and to control the potential problem patient."[6] The problem patients are dangerous and difficult; they are never happy with the results, and they sue!

As another study notes: "Even though the outcome of the cosmetic surgery is by all objective accounts successful, the patient may react, to the consternation of the surgeon, on a continuum ranging from mild dissatisfaction and requests to re-do the surgery to litigation and violence against the self or surgeon."[7] But is the purpose of the psychological test to divide those who can pass from those who, under any circumstances, are so unhappy that they will never pass? Is not the purpose of diagnosis the suggestion of treatment, rather than the refusal of treatment?

A major series of studies on the happiness of patients with the outcome of their surgery was undertaken by Meyer, Edgerton, Jacobson, and others at the Johns Hopkins University from the early 1950s to the mid-1960s. Here any abstract nature of "happiness" of the "patient" is countered by the very specific social definition of the patient population examined. A majority of these patients were Jewish, and, parallel to Freud's comment on Wittels's patient, two thirds of the women in the sample felt they had inherited their fathers' noses. This study, which framed the patients' experience by having preoperative as well as postoperative psychological testing, came to the conclusion that most found the results were favorable to the extent that they were able to modify what seemed to them an overly masculine nose.[8] Here the psychoanalytic model served as a rationale for the efficacy of the intervention. Have the father's nose reconstructed, and you remove the father from your unconscious. This is certainly a more straightforward manner of undertaking psychoanalytic psychotherapy than years of sessions on the couch. Here the efficiency of the intervention is also stressed as a substitute for psychotherapy.

The removal of the father's nose, as Freud had suggested concerning Wittels's patient, became a way of dealing with gender questions during the 1940s and 1950s. Masculinity came to be identified in the psychological literature of the 1940s and 1950s with racial identity. Thus Linn and Goldman (1949) stress that the nose became the focus of unhappiness because of anti-Semitism and xenophobia, "identification with certain culturally determined aesthetic norms," and, "probably most importantly," the nose as a "secondary sexual characteristic."[9] The link here is between the sexual identity of the unhappy rhinoplasty candidate and the cultural concept of masculinity. The right nose can represent a positive masculinity, but this masculinity comes to be normative. This is true, for Linn and Goldman, even when the patient is a woman. "Unhappiness" is defined as "believ[ing] people look down upon them because of the shape of their noses. They are shy and reclusive. In social situations they suffer from considerable anxiety" (307). Thus "two of our female patients described their feelings in almost identical words: 'There's nothing wrong with the shape of this nose,' they said, 'provided it were on a man.' One of our male patients with strong homosexual leanings drew a picture with the statement, 'This is how I'd like to look after the operation.' What he drew was the profile of a girl!" (310). The ironic response to the patient's remark marks the parallel move to the other notion of passing—here passing as a member of the "other" sex, rather than as a member of the other "race."

And yet throughout the postwar period, the overt motivation for rhinoplasty still seemed to be "ethnocultural considerations": "On a conscious level," writes the best sociologist to deal with this question, Frances Cooke Macgregor, in 1989, "prejudice and discrimination—real or imagined—and the desire to 'look American,' played a substantial role in [the patients'] motivation for surgery."[10] And indeed almost 40 percent of Macgregor's 1989 sample were Jews. In another study, Macgregor points out the radical impact of the image of the nose on patients whose own psychic makeup predisposed them to focus on their own inadequacies, hence, for example, in one case, an eighteen-year-old male student who focused on his nose, a "typically Jewish nose," as the source of his social failings.[11] While this patient was advised not to have surgery, it was clear from the detailed case description that the social environment in which he had been raised marked his nose as the appropriate focus for his status anxieties. Such patients, who see their own sense of inadequacy mirrored in the society's image of the inadequacy of the Jew, as is shown in another of Macgregor's case studies, rarely see their surgery as successful. Yet for Jews in general the level of satisfaction with rhinoplasties is higher than the norm. John M. Goin and Marcia Kraft Goin demonstrate a significantly lower index of negative responses to rhinoplasty among Jews with some 84 percent of their Jewish patients expressing a sense of the improvement of their appearance as opposed to approximately 50 percent of the other control groups.[12]

With the rise of multicultural ideas of aesthetic surgery in the 1970s and 1980s, the social category of the "ugly" begins to change. Jews are by this point more and more socialized and acculturated into American society and are no longer perceived as completely visible. They are seen as an ethnic or religious cohort rather than a racial one. The anxiety visibility is no longer keyed to the Jewish nose.[13] (But one is still anxious about being seen as "too Jewish.") Julien Reich comments in 1982, at the very beginning of this movement, that "social acceptance is also related to one's ability to fit in with the predominant group in the country in which one lives. The tremendous migratory movements induced by political and economic pressures in our time are responsible for many social problems. . . . Aesthetic plastic surgery can play an important part in helping relieve those problems related to aspects of appearance, which interfere with these aspirations."[14] Passing remains a major goal of aesthetic surgery—and indeed continues to define its psychological theory to a great degree. And passing means becoming happy with your (in)visibility.

By the close of the twentieth century, the role of "race" seems to be replaced in the psychological literature by that of "gender." However, in this reading only women have gender! It is not your visibility as an American Jew (or Italian American or African American) and your desire to pass, but rather your visibility as a "woman" that dominates the discussions of the roots of unhappiness. This seems clearly in line with the acculturation of ethnic (not racial) minorities and the rise of the women's movement.

One nonpsychoanalytic elaboration on Adler's notion of the "inferiority complex" was developed in the 1980s with the adaptation of Leon Festinger's (1919–) "theory of cognitive dissonance" for aesthetic surgery.[15] Cognitive dissonance theory provided a simple psychological mechanism to "explain" how an individual internalizes the opinions of others so that they concur with his or her own body image. Further, the classic "theory of internal self-consistency" proposed by Prescott Lecky (1892–1941) contributed the notion that any ideas that are inconsistent with one's self-image are rejected.[16] This approach emphasized the importance of "self-esteem" in defining personality structure and stressed the difference between self-perception and the perception of a specific body part. "I like me just fine," the patient says, "but I really don't like my [fill in the body part]." The qualities ascribed to the specific body part are assumed to be taken from the idealized images present in the general society, as Victor Raimy notes: "Judgments of attractive and unattractive physical appearance are social in origin."[17] Here the function of surgery is to approximate the sense of positive valence felt about the generalized self in the perception of the specific body part. In this context "unhappiness" is labeled as "discomfort." The cure is the surgical intervention in the body as well as the active reinterpretation of the categories.

Both psychotherapy and surgery complement one another in this view. What is striking is that this generalized view is seen as specifically gendered: "Female cosmetic surgery patients . . . feel less favorably toward their noses, faces, breasts than toward their overall self. These marked inconsistencies would cause 'normal' individuals to seek practical solutions of enhancing the esteem of the particular body part, to make it consistent with their general view of themselves."[18] Or "young adult females compare their level of attractiveness with that of models in ads targeted toward them causing them to indulge in unhealthy eating practices that may lead to eating disorders or to turn to invasive procedures like plastic surgery."[19] The movement toward a gendered self-consistency theory (which clearly would have worked with all early categories) was simply a complex way of discussing "passing," now understood as passing through the alteration of the internalized model of the idealized body part.

No body part is ever without symbolic meaning, and the end goal of aesthetic surgery is "to boost self-esteem" by altering the meaning ascribed to the body part. As early as 1947 Syngg and Coombs thus read aesthetic surgery as "merely" another form of psychological therapy:

> The present writer recalls a young girl with whom he once worked who was frightfully conscious of her nose. To my observation, it was not in the least unusual, but for her, it was a constant badge of shame and humiliation. Eventually, she patronized a plastic surgeon who, so she said, helped a great deal by reducing her nose, although no change was apparent to me. It was clear that she was attending to an aspect of her body directed by her concept of herself. Furthermore, a slight change in this bodily characteristic apparently resulted in considerable change in her phenomenal self.[20]

The observation of the psychologist is that the patient looks "normal." Her perception is thus pathological, and her desire to change the shape of her nose is a sign of her psychopathology. The procedure, which for the "objective" scientist makes no change in the form of the nose (and therefore obviates any "real" impact that aesthetic surgery could have had), has psychological not physical impact. Surgery thus provides a placebo function, as we have seen in the discussions of dysmorphophobia. But it is seen in terms of gender rather than ethnic identity. The desire here is to actually reconstitute the internalized image of a whole and healthy female body. It is not merely to "pass" as someone whose body is integrated or intact.

The more contemporary notion, however, that those who elect to have aesthetic surgery belong to a new class, the "disfigured," is

itself problematic. The British aesthetic surgeon Angus McGrou-
ther makes the claim that "labels such as 'morally worthy' cosmetic surgery (for burn victims) and 'morally unworthy' surgery
(seen as pandering to people's vanity)" is a false dichotomy: "Two
million people in Britain have some form of disfigurement and research suggests that plastic surgery can dramatically improve the
quality of their lives." He wishes to see all as part of the category
of the "naturally" disfigured: "We should be looking at whether
we can help people with treatment rather than whether or not it
is worthy. Someone with heart disease could have been a heavy
smoker, but someone with a disfigurement has no control over
that. We have got curious values. It's too simplistic to classify it as
life-threatening or not." The contrast with smokers is telling. They
choose to smoke (be addicted?) but no one chooses the initial shape
of his or her nose. The autonomous act of smoking is prohibited;
the autonomous act of electing surgery, praised. He continues that
"it is society at large which needs treatment. We need to adjust
our views about body image. Disfigurement is the last bastion of
discrimination." Is seeing oneself as different "disfigurement," or
is disfigurement in the eye of the beholder? Or do both reinforce
one another? If they do, the entire modern distinction between reconstructive and aesthetic surgery vanishes, which, of course, is
his point. We must not, he claims, be influenced by the culture
in which we live to see ourselves as different: "We always used to
have beautiful icons to look at but now there is encouragement
to imitate those icons." This double bind of desiring and yet ab-
horring the cultural significance of the body provides one further
elaboration on the impossibility of the distinction between reconstructive and aesthetic surgery based on any absolute definition.
"Passing" remains a primary way of understanding the power and
impact of aesthetic surgery.

Gender had been taken as a quality that, like psychopathology,
marked the potential inefficacy of rhinoplasty. R. M. Bittle argued
that "since the face is the most important physical representative
of our emotions and the nose is the most prominent part of the
face, not infrequently subconscious and unconscious personality
factors are equated with some real or imaginary anatomical defect
of the nose or face." Such complaints, following a psychoanalytic

model, are "often intimately involved in the individual's sexuality and 'identity.'" The cases of those individuals who would not be improved by elective rhinoplasty are gendered. They are "the hysterical personality, the depressed menopausal female, and the paranoid personality." While Bittle sees those patients having "external motivations (including the need to ease others), career or social ambitions, and the need to avoid cultural conflicts (e.g., avoidance of alien stereotype)" as potentially being helped ("made happy") through surgical intervention, he believes that those patients who have "internal motivation, including paranoid ideation, long standing feelings of deficiency in one's physical appearance, general inadequacy or low self-esteem in one's worth or ability, resentment of aging, or actual lack of a special identity due to conflicting parental identification" will have poor outcomes.[21] Here it is the old argument dressed in new clothes—the social conflict can be ameliorated through passing, but internal inadequacies, such as hysteria, menopause, and paranoia, mark an individual (now read: women) who cannot be helped by aesthetic surgery.

Discussions of the role of gender can be found throughout the contemporary psychological literature on aesthetic surgery. Gender (defined as the gender of the woman) plays a major role in the psychological literature on transgender and transsexual surgery as well as in the wide range of studies of the meaning of gender in the construction of the "unhappiness" of the woman and her turn to aesthetic surgery. Such surgery is seen in very contradictory ways: Aesthetic surgery is seen as a means of placing the woman in a position of power concerning her own body or is seen as making her complicit with patriarchal standards of beauty.[22] Certainly such approaches assume that the "happiness" of the female patient is either "true" (because she has taken control of her life) or "illusionary" because she is still in thrall to cultural definitions of beauty, which she can never truly acquire. These contradictions are a permanent part of the construction of the psyche as imagined in the context of contemporary aesthetic surgery.

"Self-consistency" is always defined in terms of the psyche when the psychological literature examines a patient considering aesthetic surgery. J. Burk, S. L. Zelen, and E. O. Terino examined underlying attitudes about the general self and the specific body part operated on in aesthetic surgery. They claimed that female aesthetic surgery patients would feel less favorably toward their noses, faces, or breasts than toward their overall self. These marked inconsistencies would cause "normal" individuals to seek practical solutions of enhancing the esteem of the particular body part, to make it consistent with their general view of themselves. Forty female cosmetic surgery patients were tested before and two and four months after surgery. Here the female aesthetic surgery patient is defined as a normal woman in terms of self-esteem who is attempting to remediate a consciously felt inconsistency between general and specific body-part esteem. Aesthetic surgery seems to reduce this inconsistency.[23]

Such studies run absolutely counter to those that mark gender as a source of "unhappiness," whether in terms of a biological definition of sexuality (as in postmenopausal depression) or in a cultural definition (of aesthetic surgery as the internalization of patriarchal norms). What is clear is that the model of passing that dominates the discussion of "ethnic" aesthetic surgery has simply been extended into the realm of gender. Can one undertake aesthetic surgery and "pass" unnoticed and unspoken into the realm of the "feminine"? Or does such surgery by definition mark one as subjugated to the norms of a patriarchal society? Here it is the world of the feminine represented by feminist psychologists that defines the "happy" outcome.

Thus the claims of aesthetic surgery as psychotherapy cannot stop. Once they do, the entire project of remaking the body will fall to those claiming that aesthetic surgery merely creates "false consciousness." Most recently, at the Thirtieth Anniversary Meeting of the American Society for Aesthetic Plastic Surgery, May 2–7, 1997, one of the highlights was a paper that concluded that aesthetic surgery makes patients truly happy. The press release of the organization stressed the psychotherapeutic dimension of aesthetic surgery. "The purpose of cosmetic surgery is to improve a person's psychological functioning by modifying their body image," said Gregory Borah, chief of plastic surgery at the University of Medicine and Dentistry of New Jersey–Robert Wood Johnson Medical School: "This prospective study is important because it demonstrates that objective measurements of a patient's quality of life are improved after cosmetic surgery." Borah's study involved 105 cosmetic plastic surgery patients between the ages of eighteen and seventy who answered four psychological questionnaires measuring ways of coping, personal resources, depression, and quality of life. They were completed before and after surgery. And as with Jacques Joseph's first patient, the patients showed a "significantly lower depression score at six months following surgery compared to their preoperative levels." They were also better adjusted and felt better about themselves. Such claims are necessary for the aesthetic surgeons. They counter other studies that argue that there is a marked increase in depression ("unhappiness") following aesthetic surgery. One study that relies on the reporting of nurses (rather than surgeons) noted that surgeons tended to dismiss the possibility of postoperative psychological distress and do not prepare patients well for such an outcome.[24] "Unhappiness" cannot be the outcome, except in mentally "unstable" patients, given the cultural presuppositions of aesthetic surgery. Few surgeons give much thought to the model of the mind they are evoking when they make such suppositions.

Such approaches are incorporated into the general views as to what makes for a "successful" (psychologically fulfilling) outcome for aesthetic surgery, because they claim the "restoration of an ideal state that already exists in the [patient's] imagination."[25] Aesthetic surgery does not remove psychological symptoms because there are none. This is in line with the claims that aesthetic surgery does not manufacture patients; there is no patient role and therefore the individual retains a sense of autonomy. The choice to have aesthetic surgery comes to be one that is either a product of "false consciousness" or of free will. The individual who sees himself or herself as "ugly" or defective rather than diseased is either internalizing the norms of a society of conspicuous consumption or freed from the pathologizing effect of the medicalization of appearance. The success of postadolescent rhinoplasty, which seems to have the highest success rate of all aesthetic surgical procedures, lies either in the general agreement between patient and parents concerning the transformation of the body or in the domination of the Law of the Father in defining the body of the (female) child. Unlike dieting, such procedures are passive and require no effort on the part of the client. This is understood as either the voluntary relinquishment of power or its loss. The uneventful face-lift in older women is described as part of a recuperation from traumatic emotional loss through a reinforcement of existing defenses or as the internalization of the youth cult.

These multiple, contradictory readings are the result of the ideology on the part of the group into which the aesthetic surgical patients (and surgeons) wish to be integrated. Passing is either acquiring "health" and "happiness" or being seen as "ill" and "psychopathological." Both qualities are those attributed to the individual who wishes to "pass" unnoticed.[26] Depending on how the overall effect is defined, the psyche comes to have different contours and responds to different, often contradictory therapies. Body sculpture and psychic sculpture may be closely related, but in ways that are myriad in their possibilities. Each age needs to construct or answer the way it sees aesthetic surgery functioning or not functioning as part of its conception of the body and the psyche.

Notes

PREFACE

1 Diane Coyle, "I Was So Ugly . . . ," *Independent* (March 5, 1997): 7.

2 Suzanne Harper, "A Subtle Psychology: The Perceptions and Realities of Cosmetic Surgery," *Dallas Morning News* (August 1, 1994).

3 "1996 ASPRS National Plastic Surgery Procedural," *PR Newswire* (April 28, 1997).

4 Harper.

5 Chris Martell, "For Him," *Wisconsin State Journal* (January 26, 1997): 4G.

6 See Sander L. Gilman, *The Jew's Body* (New York: Routledge, 1991), pp. 169–93.

7 Iris Krasnow, "*UPI LifeStyle:* Face lifts, Tummy Tucks, No Longer Just for Grandmothers," (October 15, 1985).

1. RECONSTRUCTING WHAT?

1 On the history of aesthetic surgery, see Otto Hildebrand, *Die Entwicklung der plastischen Chirugie* (Berlin: August Hirschwald, 1909); Karl Kassel, *Geschichte der Nasenheilkunde von ihren Anfängen bis zum 19.Jahrhundert* (1914; repr., Hildesheim: Olms, 1967); Maxwell Maltz, *Evolution of Plastic Surgery* (New York: Froben Press, 1946); George Bankoff, *The Story of Plastic Surgery* (London: Faber and Faber, 1952); Pierre-François Grigaut, *La Chirugie esthétique et plastique* (Paris: Presses Universitaires de France, 1962); Allan Ragnell, *The Development of Plastic Surgery in Stockholm in the Last Decennium* (Stockholm: Acta chirurgica Scandinavica, Supplementum 348, 1965); Frank McDowell, ed., *The McDowell Indexes of Plastic Surgical Literature*, 5 vols. (Baltimore: Williams and Wilkins, 1977–1981); McDowell, ed., *The Source Book of Plastic Surgery* (Baltimore: Williams and Wilkins, 1977); Antony F. Wallace, *The Progress of Plastic Surgery: An Intro-*

ductory History (Oxford: Willem A. Meeuws, 1982); M. Eberle, *Die Geschichte der Lippenplastik* (Ph.D. diss., Freiburg I. Br., 1982); Joachim Gabka and Ekkehard Vaubel, *Plastic Surgery, Past and Present: Origin and History of Modern Lines of Incision* (Munich: S. Karger, 1983); Mario González-Ulloa, ed., *The Creation of Aesthetic Plastic Surgery* (New York: Springer, 1985); Jerome P. Webster, "The Story of a Plastic Surgery Library," *Proceedings of the Charaka Club* 12 (1985): 14–24; Willard L. Marmelzat, "History of Dermatologic Surgery: From the Beginnings to Late Antiquity," *Clinics in Dermatology* 5 (1987): 33–43; Lenore Wright Anderson, "Synthetic Beauty: American Women and Cosmetic Surgery" (Ph.D. diss., Rice University, 1989); John Camp, *Plastic Surgery: The Kindest Cut* (New York: Henry Holt, 1989); June Thurber Cox, "Cultural Images of the Body: An Inquiry into the History of Human Engineering" (Ph.D. diss., University of California at Berkeley, 1990); D. J. Reisberg and S. W. Habakuk, "A History of Facial and Ocular Prosthetics," *Advances in Ophthalmic Plastic and Reconstructive Surgery* 8 (1990): 11–24; A. Faga and L. Valdatta, "Plastic Surgery in the Early Nineteenth Century: Notes on the Collections in the University of Pavia's Museum of History," *Plastic and Reconstructive Surgery* 86 (1990): 1220–26; Heinz-Peter Schmiedebach, Rolf Winau, and Rudolf Häring, eds., *Erste Operationen Berliner Chirugen 1817–1931* (Berlin: De Gruyter, 1990), pp. 131–78; Anne Marie Balsamo, "Reading the Gendered Body in Contemporary Culture, 1980–1990 (Body Building, Feminist Theory)" (Ph.D. diss., University of Illinois at Urbana-Champaign, 1991); B. Haeseker, "1891–1991: The Centenary of Innovative Reconstructive Hand Surgery by Carl Nicoladoni," *British Journal of Plastic Surgery* 44 (1991): 306–9; Erwin Haas, *Plastische Gesichtschirurgie* (Stuttgart: Georg Thieme Verlag, 1991); August Lange, "Die Rhinoplastik im 'Goettingischen Taschenkalender auf das Jahr 1805': Eine Bemerkung zur Geschichte der Nasenwiederherstellung," *Würzburger medizinhistorische Mitteilungen* 9 (1991): 345–50; Robert Scheer, *The Cosmetic Surgery Revolution: An Objective Guide to Understanding Your Cosmetic Surgery Choices* (Los Angeles: Summit Pines Press, 1992); M. Bernklau, *Über die historischen Entwicklung der rekonstruktiven Gesichtschirugie in der Zeit von 1800 bis 1950* (Ph.D. diss., Giessen, 1992); A. C. Elias, "A Case of Cheiloplasty—1864," *Journal of Oral and Maxillofacial Surgery* 50 (1992): 998–99; Sharon Romm, *The Changing Face of Beauty* (St. Louis, Mo.: Mosby Year Book, 1992); Willard L. Marmelzat, "Bits of History, Bits of Mystery: A Historical Review of Chemical Rejuvenation of the Face," in Robert Kotler, ed., *Chemical Rejuvenation of the Face* (St. Louis, Mo.: Mosby Year Book, 1992): 33–39; Noëlle Châtelet, *Trompe-l'oeil: Voyage au pays de la chi-*

rurgie esthétique (Paris: Belfond, 1993); Kurt Kristen, "Zur Geschichte der Kieferchirugie dargestellt am Beispiel der Rehabiliationen von Trägern einer Lippen-Kiefer-Gaumenspalte," *Sitzungsberichte der Heidelberger Akademie der Wissenschaften* (1993–1994): 33–47; Albino Comelli, *Da narciso al narcisismo: Storia e psicologia del corpo: Costume, medicina, estetica* (Trento: Reverdito, 1993); David M. Reifler, ed., *The American Society of Ophthalmic Plastic and Reconstructive Surgery (ASOPRS): The First Twenty-Five Years: 1969–1994: History of Ophthalmic Plastic Surgery: 2500 BC–AD 1994* (Winter Park, Fla.: American Society of Ophthalmic Plastic and Reconstructive Surgery, 1994); Peter Proff, "Möglichkeiten der Plastisch-Rekonstruktiven und Tumor-Chirurgie in der frühbyzantinischen Medizin," in Josef Domes et al., eds., *Licht der Natur: Medizin in Fachliteratur und Dichtung* (Göppingen: Kummerle, 1994), pp. 307–28; Christoph Weisser, "Die Nasenersatzplastik nach Heinrich von Pfalzpaint: Ein Beitrag zur Geschichte der plastischen Chirurgie im Spätmittelalter mit Edition des Textes," in Domes et al., pp. 485–506; Elizabeth G. Haiken, "Body and Soul: Plastic Surgery in the United States, 1914–1990," (Ph.D. diss., University of California, Berkeley, 1994); Elizabeth G. Haiken, "Plastic Surgery and American Beauty in 1921," *Bulletin of the History of Medicine* 68 (1994): 429–53; M. G. H. Bishop, "The Making and Re-making of Man 1: Mary Shelley's 'Frankenstein' and Transplant Surgery," *Journal of the Royal Society of Medicine* 87 (1994): 749–51; Kathy Davis, *Reshaping the Female Body: The Dilemma of Cosmetic Surgery* (New York: Routledge, 1995); S. Furlan and R. F. Mazzola, "Alessandro Benedetti, a Fifteenth Century Anatomist and Surgeon: His Role in the History of Nasal Reconstruction," *Plastic and Reconstructive Surgery* 96 (1995): 739–43; Walter Hoffmann-Axthelm et al., *Die Geschichte der Mund-,Kiefer-und Gesichtschirurgie* (Berlin: Quintessenz Verag, 1995); Anne Balsamo, *Technologies of the Gendered Body: Reading Cyborg Women* (Durham, N.C.: Duke University Press, 1996); Peter Paul Brunner, *Die Entwicklung der Knochenplastik am Unterkiefer im Ersten Weltkrieg* (Zurich: Juris, 1996). Following the completion of this manuscript a revision of Elizabeth Haiken's excellent study of aesthetic surgery in the United States appeared under the title of *Venus Envy: A History of Cosmetic Surgery* (Baltimore: Johns Hopkins University Press, 1997). Her altered title points toward a focus on gender that is, however, not the center of her work. See also the recent essay by Kathy Davis, "Pygmalions in Plastic Surgery," *Health* 2 (1998): 23–40.

2   Frederick Strange Kolle, *Plastic and Cosmetic Surgery* (New York: D. Appleton, 1911), p. 339.

3   Harold Gillies and D. Ralph Millard, *The Principles and Art of Plastic*

Surgery, 2 vols. (Boston: Little, Brown [1957]), 1: 32. See also Gillies's earlier comments in his Charles H. Mayo lecture for 1934, *The Development and Scope of Plastic Surgery* (Chicago: Northwestern University Press, 1935).

4 Gustavo Sanvenero-Rosselli, *Chirurgia plastica del naso* (Rome: Pozzi, 1931), p. 34.

5 Mary Sharon Webb, "Beyond Beauty: Philosophy, Ethics and Plastic Surgery" (Ph.D. diss., Yale University, 1984).

6 On the beauty myth, see Gerald R. Adams and Sharyn M. Crossman, *Physical Attractiveness: A Cultural Imperative* (Roslyn Heights, NY: Libra, 1978); Lois W. Banner, *American Beauty* (Chicago: University of Chicago Press, 1983); Robin Tolmach Lakoff and Raquel L. Scherr, *Face Value: The Politics of Beauty* (Routledge and Kegan Paul, 1984); Hillel Schwartz, *Never Satisfied: A Cultural History of Diets, Fantasies, and Fat* (New York: Free Press, 1986); Wendy Chapkis, *Beauty Secrets: Women and the Politics of Appearance* (Boston: South End Press, 1986); Sabra Waldfogel, "The Body Beautiful, the Body Hateful: Feminine Body Image and the Culture of Consumption in 20th-Century America" (Ph.D. diss., University of Minnesota, 1986); Arthur Marwick, *Beauty in History: Society, Politics, and Personal Appearance* (London: Thames and Hudson, 1988); Camille Paglia, *Sexual Personae: Art and Decadence from Nefertiti to Emily Dickinson* (New Haven: Yale University Press, 1990); Naomi Wolf, *The Beauty Myth: How Images of Beauty Are Used against Women* (New York: W. Morrow, 1991); Sara Halprin, *Look at My Ugly Face: Myths and Musings on Beauty and Other Perilous Obsessions with Women's Appearance* (New York: Viking, 1995); Kaz Cooke, *Real Gorgeous: The Truth about Body and Beauty* (London: Bloomsbury, 1995); Efrat Tseëlon, *The Masque of Femininity: The Presentation of Woman in Everyday Life* (London: Sage, 1995); Nancy Friday, *The Power of Beauty* (New York: Harper Collins, 1996); Richard Sartore, *Body Shaping: Trends, Fashions, and Rebellions* (Commack, N.Y.: Nova Science Publishers, 1996); Frida Kerner Furman, *Facing the Mirror: Older Women and Beauty Shop Culture* (New York: Routledge, 1997).

7 Hans-Peter Wengle, "The Psychology of Cosmetic Surgery: A Critical Overview of the Literature 1960–1982," *Annals of Plastic Surgery* 16 (1986): 435.

8 Cited by Robert M. Goldwyn, *The Patient and the Plastic Surgeon* (Boston: Little, Brown, 1991), p. 52.

9 Neil Shulman, *What? Dead Again? A Novel* (Baton Rouge, La.: Legacy, 1979).

10   On the history of the representation of aesthetic surgery in the cinema see Stuart C. Callé and James T. Evans, "Plastic Surgery in the Cinema, 1917–1993," *Plastic and Reconstructive Surgery* 93 (1994): 422–33.

11   "1996 ASPRS National Plastic Surgery Procedural."

12   John M. Graham Jr., *Smith's Recognizable Patterns of Human Deformation* (Philadelphia: W. B. Saunders, 1988), p. 1.

13   W. Rosenthal, "The Disfigured Man and His Psyche," *Aesthetica* 2 (1961): 6–7.

14   See the discussion in Walter E. Kunstler, "Aesthetic Considerations in Surgical Operations from Antiquity to Recent Times," *Bulletin of the History of Medicine* 12 (1942): 27–69.

15   The translation from the Edwin Smith Papyrus on the fracture of the nose is reprinted in McDowell, *Source Book*, pp. 54–64.

16   Aulus Cornelius Celsus, *De medicina*, trans. and intro. by W. G. Spence, 3 vols. (Cambridge, Mass.: Harvard University Press, 1935–1938), 3: 339.

17   Erich Lexer, *Wiederherstellungschirurgie* (Leipzig: Johann Ambrosius Barth, 1920), pp. 62–63.

18   Thom Jones, *Cold Snap: Stories* (Boston: Little, Brown, 1995), pp. 120–46.

19   Ricardo Baroudi, "Why Aesthetic Plastic Surgery Became Popular in Brazil?" *Plastic Surgery* 27 (1991): 396.

20   Marsha L. Vanderford and David H. Smith, *The Silicone Breast Implant Story* (Mahwah, N.J.: Lawrence Erlbaum, 1996), p. 25.

21   André Jean Marie Goumain and Alexianne G. Izquierdo, *De Quelques Aspects sociaux psychologiques et psychiatriques de la chirurgie esthètique* (Paris: Odéon, 1957), p. 4.

2. PSYCHIC PAIN

1   On the psychological and social construction of the body, see Stephen Kern, *Anatomy and Destiny: A Cultural History of the Human Body* (Indianapolis, Ind.: Bobbs-Merrill, 1975); Jean Maisonneuve and Marilou Bruchon-Schweitzer, *Modeles du corps et psychologie esthétique* (Paris: Presses Universitaires de France, 1981); Pedro Laín-Entralgo, *El cuerpo humano* (Madrid: Espasa Calpe, 1987); Marilou Bruchon-Schweitzer, *Une Psychologie du corps* (Paris: Presses Universitaires de France, 1990); Barbara Duden, *The Woman Beneath the Skin: A Doctor's Patients in Eighteenth-Century Germany*, trans. Thomas Dunlap (Cambridge, Mass.: Harvard University Press, 1991); Jon Stratton, *The Desirable Body: Cultural Fetishism and the Erotics of Consumption* (Manchester: Manchester University Press, 1996); Susan Bordo, *Twi-*

light Zones: The Hidden Life of Cultural Images from Plato to O.J. (Berkeley: University of California Press, 1997).

2   Sue Arnold, "On the Radio: Not Far from the Madding Cows," *Observer* (December 10, 1995): 17.

3   "Technological Advances Lead Many to Undergo Smaller Procedures in Facial Plastic Surgery, New Survey Shows," *PR Newswire* (October 8, 1996).

4   *New York Times* (March 11, 1937): 25. On Crum, see Haiken, *Body and Soul*, pp. 120–26.

5   "New Bodies for Sale," *Newsweek* (May 27, 1985): 64–71.

6   Edward Shorter, *From Paralysis to Fatigue: A History of Psychosomatic Illness in the Modern Era* (New York: Free Press, 1993), and Shorter, *From the Mind into the Body: The Cultural Origins of Psychosomatic Symptoms* (New York: Free Press, 1994). Sander L. Gilman, *The Case of Sigmund Freud: Medicine and Identity at the Fin de Siècle* (Baltimore: Johns Hopkins University Press, 1993), and Gilman, *Freud, Race, and Gender* (Princeton: Princeton University Press, 1993).

7   Sigmund Freud, *Standard Edition of the Complete Psychological Works of Sigmund Freud*, ed. and trans., J. Strachey et al., 24 vols. (London: Hogarth, 1955–1974), 2: 305. All subsequent quotations from Freud's works in this study are from this edition, referred to in the notes as SE.

8   SE 3: 143.

9   See, for example, Peter C. Olley's summary of the standard indications for negative outcome in his essay "Psychiatric Aspects of Cosmetic Surgery," in John G. Howells, ed., *Modern Perspective in the Psychiatric Aspects of Surgery* (New York: Brunner/Mazel, 1976), pp. 508–9.

10 SE 7: 16–17 n. 2. My interpretations of Freud's reading of the case of Dora have appeared in *Difference and Pathology: Stereotypes of Sexuality, Race, and Madness* (Ithaca, NY: Cornell University Press, 1985), pp. 182–84, and *The Jew's Body*, pp. 81–89.

11 See Sander L. Gilman, "Why Is Schizophrenia 'Bizarre': An Historical Essay in the Vocabulary of Psychiatry," *Journal of the History of the Behavioral Sciences* 19 (1983): 127–35.

12 Sanford Gifford, "Cosmetic Surgery and Personality Change: A Review and Some Clinical Operations," in Robert M. Goldwyn, ed., *The Unfavorable Result in Plastic Surgery: Avoidance and Treatment* (Boston: Little, Brown, 1972), pp. 11–33.

13 Carl Gustav Carus, *Psyche: Zur Entwicklungsgeschichte der Seele* (Pforzheim: Flammer und Hoffmann, 1846), p. 56.

14 Franz Alexander, *The Medical Value of Psychoanalysis* (New York: Norton, 1936).

15 Friedrich Curtius, *Konstitution und Vererbung in der klinischen Medizin* (Berlin: A. Metzner, 1935), and Curtius, *Moderne Asthmabehandlung: Atemschulung, Entspannung, Psychotherapie* (Berlin: Springer-Verlag, 1965).

16 Mary Douglas, *Natural Symbols* (New York: Pantheon, 1970), p. 70.

17 Octavio Paz, "Eroticism and Gastrosophy," *Daedalus* 101 (1972): 77.

18 Henry J. Schireson, *As Others See You: The Story of Plastic Surgery* (New York: Macaulay, 1938), p. vii.

19 Gloria Anzaldúa, *Borderlands/La Frontera: The New Mestiza* (San Francisco: Aunt Lute Books, 1987), p. 3.

3. THE MEDICALIZATION OF AESTHETIC SURGERY

1   Jonathan Friedland, "Argentina Is a Land of Many Faces, Fixed by Plastic Surgeons," *Wall Street Journal* (February 2, 1996): 1.

2   Richard Sennett, *The Fall of Public Man* (New York: Norton, 1974), p. 70.

3   Lewis Mumford, *The Myth of the Machine: Techniques and Human Development* (New York: Harcourt, Brace, and World, 1967), p. 109.

4   Charles Darwin, *The Descent of Man and Selection in Relation to Sex* (New York: D. Appelton, 1897), p. 575.

5   Philip Cassell, ed., *The Giddens Reader* (Stanford, Calif.: Stanford University Press, 1993), p. 304.

6   Christopher Derek Kenway, "Kraft und Schönheit: Regeneration and Racial Theory in the German Physical Culture Movement, 1895–1920," (Ph.D. diss., University of California at Los Angeles, 1996).

7   Kolle, pp. 190–91.

8   Methodologically I am following the approach of Klaus Müller, *Aber in meinem Herzen Sprach eine Stimme so laut: Homosexuelle Autobiographien und medizinische Pathographien im neunzehnten Jahrhundert* (Berlin: Verlag Rosa Winkel, 1991), on homosexual narratives in Imperial medical texts.

4. A BEAUTIFUL BODY IS A HAPPY MIND

1   SE 2: 305.

2   Luis Majul, *Las mascaras de la Argentina: Cambios esteticos, patrimoniales, psicologicos e ideologicos de los argentinos que estan en la vidriera* (Buenos Aires: Atlantida, 1995).

3   Susanna Stolz, *Die Handwerke der Körpers: Bäder, Barbier, Perückenmacher, Friseur: Folge und Ausdruck historischen Körperverständnisses* (Marburg: Jonas, 1992).

4   Christine E. Jones and Beulah D. Jones, "Cosmetic Surgery of the Face," *New York State Journal of Medicine* 77 (1977): 2292–93.

5   Michael Selz, "Dallas Lender Capitalizes on the Public's Yen for Uninsured Cosmetic Surgery," *Wall Street Journal* (January 15, 1997): A1.

6   Alison Boshoff and Lydia Slater, "The Remoulding of Paula," *Daily Mail* (London) (July 15, 1995): 3.

7   Nury Vittachi, "Something for the Nail-Biters to Chew on," *South China Morning Post* (May 1, 1996): 12.

8   Sarah Tippit, "Dr. Leonard Levine; Making Bodies More Perfect Makes Him Happy," *Orlando Sentinel* (April 17, 1994): 6.

9   Julien Reich, "Aesthetic Judgment in the Surgery of Appearance," *Aesthetic Plastic Surgery* 1 (1976): 40.

10 John M. Goin and Marcia Kraft Goin, *Changing the Body: Psychological Effects of Plastic Surgery* (Baltimore: Williams and Wilkins, 1981), p. 110.

11 Sennett, p. 90.

12 Adalbert G. Bettman, "The Psychology of Appearances," *Northwest Medicine* 28 (1929): 182.

13 On the history of happiness, see Stephen A. White, *Sovereign Virtue: Aristotle on the Relation between Happiness and Prosperity* (Stanford, Calif.: Stanford University Press, 1992); Maximilian Forschner, *Über das Glück des Menschen: Aristoteles, Epikur, Stoa, Thomas von Aquin, Kant* (Darmstadt: Wissenschaftliche Buchgesellschaft, 1993); Danielle Büschinger, ed., *L'Idée de bonheur au Moyên Age: Actes du colloque d'Amiens de mars 1984* (Göppingen: Kümmerle, 1990); Jan Lewis, *The Pursuit of Happiness, Family and Values in Jefferson's Virginia* (Cambridge: Cambridge University Press, 1983); Alan O. Ebenstein, *The Greatest Happiness Principle: An Examination of Utilitarianism* (New York: Garland, 1991).

14 John Stuart Mill, *Utilitarianism*, ed. G. Sher (Indianapolis, Ind.: Hacket, 1979), p. 7.

15 Jeremy Bentham, *An Introduction to the Principles of Morals and Legislation*, ed. J. H. Burns and H. L. A. Hart (London: Athlone Press, 1970), p. 12.

16 Ambrose Bierce, *The Devil's Dictionary*, vol. 7 of *Collected Works* (New York: Neale Publishing Company, 1911), p. 130.

17 Leon Kass, *Toward a More Natural Science: Biology and Human Affairs* (New York: Free Press, 1984), p. 160.

18 Aristotle, *Physiognomics, The Complete Works of Aristotle*, 2 vols., ed. Jonathan Barnes (Princeton: Princeton University Press, 1984), 1: 1238.

19 Charles Siebert, "The Cuts That Go Deeper," *New York Times Maga-*

zine (July 7, 1996): 20. On Rosen, see Mark Dery, *Escape Velocity: Cyberculture at the End of the Century* (New York: Grove Press, 1996).

20 Elaine Scarry, *The Body in Pain: The Making and Unmaking of the World* (1985; repr., New York: Oxford University Press, 1987), p. 14.

5. THE PHANTOM OF THE OPÉRA'S NOSE

1 All quotations are from Gaston Leroux, *The Phantom of the Opera*, intro. Max Byrd (New York: New American Library, 1987), p. 9. See also the discussion in Slavoj Žižek, "Grimaces of the Real; or, When the Phallus Appears," *October* 58 (1991): 45–68; and Hinrich Hudde, "Ödipus als Detektive: Die Urszene als Geheimnis des geschlossenen Raums," *Zeitschrift für französische Sprache und Literatur* 86 (1976): 1–25.

2 *The Works of Voltaire*, vol. 1, *Candide* (Akron: Werner, 1904), pp. 73–74. See Jean Sareil, "Sur la génealogie de la verole," *Teaching Language through Literature* 26 (1986): 3–8.

3 Edmund About, *Le nez d'un notaire* (Paris: Calmann-Lévy, 1862).

4 Cited from Johann Friedrich Dieffenbach, *Chirurgische Erfahrungen, besonders über die Wiederherstellung zerstörter Theile des menschlichen Körpers nach neuen Methoden*, 4 vols. in 3 and atlas (Berlin: Enslin, 1829–34), 3: 39.

5 Ashley Montagu, *The Elephant Man: A Study in Human Dignity* (New York: Outerbridge and Dienstfrey, 1971); Michael Howell, *The True History of the Elephant Man* (London: Allison and Busby, 1980); Peter W. Graham, *Articulating the Elephant Man: Joseph Merrick and His Interpreters* (Baltimore: Johns Hopkins University Press, 1992).

6 Robert Gersuny, "Über einige kosmetische Operationen," *Wiener medizinische Wochenschrift* 53 (1903): 2253. On Billroth and Gersuny, see Erna Lesky, "Die Entwicklung der wissenschaftlichen Kosmetik in Österreich," *Ästhetische Medizin* 9 (1960): 199–210.

7 All references are to Marc Scott Zicree, *The Twilight Zone Companion* (Beverly Hills, Calif.: Sillman-James Press, 1992), pp. 144–49.

8 Whitley Strieber, *Communion: A True Story* (New York: Beech Tree Books, 1987).

9 Patrick Mott, "Galactic Glastnost; Trends: Extraterrestrial Beings Have Recaptured the Public Imagination—And Not Just in the United States," *Los Angeles Times* (October 26, 1989): E1.

10 Edward Dolnick, "Closer Encounters," *The New Republic* 197 (August 10, 1987): 15.

11 James S. Gordon, "The UFO Experience," *The Atlantic Monthly* 268 (August, 1991): 82.

6. THE ROLE OF AESTHETICS IN CREATING THE PSYCHE

1 Darwin, p. 585. See also John V. Pickstone, "Bureaucracy, Liberalism and the Body in post-Revolutionary France: Bichat's Physiology and the Paris school of Medicine," *History of Science* 19 (1981): 115–42, as well as C. Heywood, "D. H. Lawrence's 'Blood Consciousness' and the Work of Xavier Bichat and Marshall Hall," *Études Anglaises, Grande-Bretagne-États-Unis* 32 (1979): 397–413.

2 Karl Rosenkranz, *Ästhetik des Häßlichen* (1853; repr., Leipzig: Reclam, 1990), pp. 5–8.

3 Georges Canguilhem, *The Normal and the Pathological*, trans. Carolyn R. Fawcett (Boston: Zone, 1989).

4 Anthony Synnott, "Truth and Goodness, Mirrors and Masks: A Sociology of Beauty and the Face," *British Journal of Sociology* 40 (1989): 607–36.

5 Empedocles, Fragment 126, in Hermann Diels and Walther Kranz, eds., *Die Fragmente der Vorsokratiker, griechisch und deutsch*, 3 vols. (Berlin: Weidmann, 1951–1952), 1: 362.

6 Immanuel Kant, *The Critique of Judgment*, trans. J. C. Meredith (Oxford: Oxford University Press, 1986), p. 103. I am indebted to Jonathan Sinclair Carey, "Kant and the Cosmetic Surgeon," *Journal of the Florida Medical Association* 76 (1989): 637–43, as well as Carey, "The Quasimodo Complex: Deformity Reconsidered," *Journal of Clinical Ethics* 1 (1990): 212–36.

7 Immanuel Kant, *Werke*, 10 vols., ed. Wilhelm Weischedel (Darmstadt: Wissenschaftliche Buchgesellschaft, 1975), 8: 283–87.

8 Daniel Kevles, *In the Name of Eugenics* (New York: Alfred A. Knopf, 1985), p. 12; see also Cynthia Eagle Russett, *Sexual Science* (Cambridge, Mass.: Harvard University Press, 1989), pp. 78–92.

9 Michel Foucault, *An Introduction*, vol. 1 of *The History of Sexuality*, trans. Robert Hurley (New York: Vintage, 1980), p. 146.

10 Jules Héricourt, *The Social Diseases: Tuberculosis, Syphilis, Alcoholism, Sterility*, trans. with a final chapter by Bernard Miall (London, 1920), pp. 244–45.

11 Cicero, *Tusculan Disputations*, trans. J. E. King, Loeb Library, no. 14 (New York: G. P. Putnam's Sons, 1927), pp. 90–93.

12 J. C. Lavater, *Essays on Physiognomy* (London: B. Blake, 1840), p. 99. The most recent comprehensive introduction to Lavater is Ellis Shookman, ed., *The Faces of Physiognomy: Interdisciplinary Approaches to Johann Caspar Lavater* (Columbia, S.C.: Camden House, 1993). See also Karl Maurer, "Entstaltung: Ein beinahe untergegangener Goethescher Begriff," in Rudolf Behrens and Roland Galle, eds., *Leib-Zeichen: Kör-*

perbilder, Rhetorik und Anthropologie im 18. Jahrhundert (Würzburg: Königshausen & Neumann, 1993), pp. 151–62; Liliane Weissberg, "Literatur als Representationsform: Zur Lektüre von Lektüre," in Lutz Danneberg, et al., eds., *Vom Umgang mit Literatur und Literaturgeschichte: Positionen und Perspektive* (Stuttgart: Metzler, 1992), pp. 293–313; Richard Grey, "Die Geburt des Genies aus dem Geiste der Aufklarung: Semiotik und Aufklärungsideologie in der Physiognomik Johann Kaspar Lavaters," *Poetica* 23 (1991): 95–138, as well as Grey, "Sign and Sein: The *Physiognomikstreit* and the Dispute over the Semiotic Constitution of Bourgeois Individuality," *Deutsche Vierteljahrsschrift für Literaturwissenschaft und Geistesgeschichte* 66 (1992): 300–332; Michael Shortland, "Barthes, Lavater and the Legible Body," in Mike Gane, ed., *Ideological Representation and Power in Social Relations: Literary and Social Theory* (London: Routledge, 1989), pp. 17–53, as well as Shortland, "The Power of a Thousand Eyes: Johann Caspar Lavater's Science of Physiognomical Perception," *Criticism* 28 (1986): 379–408. Of central importance is the work of Barbara Maria Stafford, "'Peculiar Marks': Lavater and the Countenance of Blemished Thought," *Art Journal* 46 (1987): 185–92. See also Stafford, *Good Looking: Essays on the Virtue of Images* (Cambridge, Mass.: MIT Press, 1996); *Artful Science: Enlightenment, Entertainment, and the Eclipse of Visual Education* (Cambridge, Mass.: MIT Press, 1994), and *Body Criticism: Imaging the Unseen in Enlightenment Art and Medicine* (Cambridge, Mass.: MIT Press, 1991).

13   An excellent overview of this question from the standpoint of earlier theories of medical physiognomy is Barbara M. Stafford, John La Puma, and David L. Schiedermayer, "One Face of Beauty, One Picture of Health: The Hidden Aesthetic of Medical Practice," *Journal of Medicine and Philosophy* 14 (1989): 213–30.

14   See George L. Mosse, *Toward the Final Solution: A History of European Racism* (New York: H. Fertig, 1978), and, on Winckelmann's impact throughout European culture, Joan DeJean, *Fictions of Sappho 1546–1937* (Chicago: University of Chicago Press, 1989), pp. 206–7.

15   Friedrich Nietzsche, *The Genealogy of Morals*, trans. Francis Golffing (New York: Doubleday, 1956), pp. 167–68.

16   Immanuel Kant, *Observations of the Feeling of the Beautiful and Sublime*, trans. John T. Goldthwait (Berkeley: University of California Press, 1960), p. 87.

17   Barbara Freeman, "The Rise of the Sublime: Sacrifice and Misogyny in Eighteenth-Century Aesthetics," *Yale Journal of Criticism* 4 (1992): 81–99.

18   Anatole Leroy-Beaulieu, *Israel among the Nations: A Study of the Jews*

and Antisemitism, trans. Frances Hellman (New York: G. P. Putnam's Sons, 1895), p. 247. All subsequent references are to this translation. The book was first published as Anatole Leroy-Beaulieu, that is, Henry Jean Baptiste Anatole, *Les Juifs et l'antisémitisme: Israél chez les nations* (Paris: Lévy, 1893), which went through at least seven printings in 1893 alone. Of his other works, see *La Révolution et le libéralisme: Essais de critique et d'histoire* (Paris: Hachette, 1890), and the pamphlet *Les Immigrants juifs et le judäisme aux États-Unis* (Paris: Librairie nouvelle, 1905). On his work, see Martha Helms Cooley, "Nineteenth-Century French Historical Research on Russia: Louis Leger, Alfred Rambaud, Anatole Leroy-Beaulieu" (Ph.D. diss., Indiana University, 1971).

19 Sander L. Gilman, *Difference and Pathology: Stereotypes of Sexuality, Race, and Madness* (Ithaca, NY: Cornell University Press, 1985), pp. 76–109.

20 Richard Burke, *A Historical Chronology of Tuberculosis* (Springfield, IL: C. C. Thomas, 1938), p. 17.

21 Max Neuburger, "Zur Geschichte der Konstitutionslehre," *Zeitschrift für angewandte Anatomie und Konstitutionslehre* 1 (1914): 4–10.

1. JOHN ORLANDO ROE'S PRAGMATIC PSYCHOLOGY

1 J. F. Dieffenbach, *Die operative Chirugie*, 2 vols. (Leipzig: Brockhaus, 1845), 1: 312–92 on plastic surgery of the nose. See also Richard Lampe, *Dieffenbach* (Leipzig: J. A. Barth, 1934); Wolfgang Genschorek, *Wegbereiter der Chirurgie: Johann Friedrich Dieffenbach, Theodor Billroth* (Leipzig: S. Hirzel, 1982); U. Ulrich and C. Lauritzen, "Johann Friedrich Dieffenbach, 1792–1847: 'Vater der plastischen Chirurgie' in Deutschland," *Deutsche medizinische Wochenschrift* 117 (1992): 1165–67; F. E. Mueller, "Der Chirurg Johann Friedrich Dieffenbach und sein Einfluss auf die Entwicklung der Plastischen Chirurgie," *Chirurgie* 63 (1992): 127–31; H. Wolff, "Das chirurgische Erbe: Zum 200. Geburtstag von Johann Friedrich Dieffenbach," *Zentralblatt für Chirurgie* 117 (1992): 238–43. On the institutional history of reconstructive surgery in Berlin, see Paul Diepgen and Paul Rostock, eds., *Das Universitätsklinikum in Berlin: Seine Ärzte und seine wissenschaftliche Leistung* (Leipzig: Barth, 1939), pp. 66–80 on Dieffenbach, pp. 55–66 on Graefe; and Gerhard Jaeckel, *Die Charité: Die Geschichte eines Weltzentrums der Medizin* (Bayreuth: Hestia, 1963), pp. 231, 238–47 on Graefe and Dieffenbach.

2 John O. Roe, "The Deformity Termed 'Pug Nose' and Its Correction,

by a Simple Operation," *Medical Record* 31 (June 4, 1887): 621–23; repr. in McDowell, *Source Book*, p. 114. See Blair O. Rogers, "John Orlando Roe—Not Jacques Joseph—the Father of Aesthetic Rhinoplasty," *Aesthetic Plastic Surgery* 10 (1986): 63–88.

3   John O. Roe, "The Correction of Nasal Deformities," in McDowell, *Source Book*, p. 3.

4   Robert F. Weir, "On Restoring Sunken Noses without Scarring the Face," *New York Medical Journal* 56 (1892): 449–54, cited in McDowell, *Source Book*, p. 141.

5   Jacques Joseph, "Operative Reduction of the Size of a Nose (Rhinomiosis)," trans. Gustave Aufricht, *Plastic and Reconstructive Surgery* 46 (1970): 178; repr. in McDowell, *Source Book*, pp. 164–67. The essay was originally published as "Über die operative Verkleinerung einer Nase (Rhinomiosis)," *Berliner klinische Wochenschrift* 40 (1898): 882–85. See also Paul Natvig, *Jacques Joseph: Surgical Sculptor* (Philadelphia: W. B. Saunders, 1982), pp. 23–24. See also C. Walter and D. J. Brain, "Jacques Joseph," *Facial Plastic Surgery* 9 (1993): 116–24; S. Milstein, "Jacques Joseph and the Upper Lateral Nasal Cartilages," *Plastic and Reconstructive Surgery* 78 (1986): 424; D. J. Hauben, "Jacques Joseph (1865–1934)," *Laryngologie, Rhinologie, Otologie* 62 (1983): 56–57; T. Gibson and D. W. Robinson, "The Mammary Artery Pectoral Flaps of Jacques Joseph," *British Journal of Plastic Surgery* 29 (1976): 370–76; Paul Natvig, "Some Aspects of the Character and Personality of Jacques Joseph," *Plastic and Reconstructive Surgery* 47 (1971): 452–53. On the general history of rhinoplasty, see Blair O. Rogers, "A Chronological History of Cosmetic Surgery," *Bulletin of the New York Academy of Medicine* 47 (1971): 265–302; Blair O. Rogers, "A Brief History of Cosmetic Surgery," *Surgical Clinics of North America* 51 (1971): 265–88; H. Rudert, "Von der submukosen Septumresektion Killians uber Cottles Septumplastik zur modernen plastischen Septumkorrektur und funktionellen Septo-Rhinoplastik," *Hals-Nase-Ohren* 32 (1984): 230–33; D. J. Hauben, "Die Geschichte der Rhinoplastik," *Laryngologie, Rhinologie, Otologie* 62 (1983): 53–55; P. A. Adamson, "Rhinoplasty—Our Past," *Facial Plastic Surgery* 5 (1988): 93–96; C. Walter, "The Evolution of Rhinoplasty," *Journal of Laryngology and Otology* 102 (1988): 1079–85; I. Eisenberg, "A History of Rhinoplasty," *South African Medical Journal* 62 (1982): 286–92; A. B. Sokol and R. B. Berggren, "Rhinoplasty: Its Development and Present Day Usages," *Ohio State Medical Journal* 68 (1972): 556–62.

6   Joseph, "Operative Reduction," p. 180.

7   Jacques Joseph, "Nasenverkleinerung (mit Krankenvorstellung)," *Deutsche Medizinische Wochenschrift* 30 (1904): 1095. See also Joseph,

"Nasenverkleinerungen," *Verhandlungen der deutsche Gesellschaft für Chirugie* 33 (1904): 112–20, as well as Joseph, *Eine Nasenplastik, ausgeführt in Lokalanesthesie* (Berlin: G. Stilke, 1927).

8   N. J. Knorr, M. T. Edgerton, and J. E. Hoopes, "The 'Insatiable' Cosmetic Surgery Patient," *Plastic and Reconstructive Surgery* 40 (1967): 285–89.

9   Jean-Jacques Rousseau, *Oeuvres complètes*, ed. V. D. Musset-Pathay, 4 vols. (Paris: F. Didot, 1823), 3: 20.

10   Alfred Berndorfer, "Aesthetic Surgery as Organopsychic Therapy," *Aesthetic and Plastic Surgery* 3 (1979): 143. For a good critique of this problem, see David A. Hyman, "Aesthetics and Ethics: The Implications of Cosmetic Surgery," *Perspectives in Biology and Medicine* 33 (1990): 190–202.

11   Lewis Perry Curtis, *Apes and Angels: The Irishman in Victorian Caricature* (Washington, DC: Smithsonian Institution Press, 1971). For images of jaws and noses see pp. 20f., 29f., 45.

2. ENRICO MORSELLI'S DYSMORPHOPHOBIA

1   This discussion is indebted to M. Vanini and G. Weiss, "Contributo clinico allo studio dei disturbi della corporeitá psicotica," *Revista sperimentale di freniatria e medicine legale della alienzioni mentali* 96 (1972): 32–55; Katharine A. Phillips, "Body Dysmorphic Disorder: The Distress of Imagined Ugliness," *American Journal of Psychiatry* 148 (1991): 1138–49; German E. Berrios, *The History of Mental Symptoms: Descriptive Psychopathology since the Nineteenth Century* (Cambridge: Cambridge University Press, 1996), pp. 276–81.

2   Enrico Morselli, "Sulla dismorfofobia e sulla tefefobia: Due forme non per anco de scritte di Pazzia con idee fisse," *Bolletinno dell r. accademia di Genova* 6 (1891): 110–19.

3   Nancy Stepan, *The Idea of Race in Science: Great Britain, 1800–1960* (London: Macmillan, in association with St. Anthony's College, Oxford, 1982), p. 103.

4   Paolo Mantegazza, *Physiognomy and Expression* (London: W. Scott, 1904), p. 45.

5   Theodor Meynert, "Über Zwangsvorstellungen," *Wiener klinische Wochenschrift* 77 (1888): 109–12, 139–41, 170–72.

6   Richard Krafft-Ebing, *Nervosität und Neurasthenische Zustände* (Vienna: Alfred Hölder, 1895), p. 54. (This was also published as part of vol. 12 of Hermann Nothnagel, ed., *Specielle Pathologie und Therapie*, 24 vols. [Vienna: Alfred Hölder, 1894–1908].)

7   Emil Kraepelin, "Zur Entartungsfrage," *Zentralblatt für Nervenheilkunde und Psychiatrie* 19 (1908): 748.

8   Emil Kraepelin, *Psychiatrie,* 8th ed., 4 vols. (Leipzig: J. A. Barth, 1909–1915), vol. 4, pt. 3, p. 1861.

9   Docteur Celticus, *Les 19 Tares corporelles visibles pour reconnaitre un juif* (Paris: Librairie Antisemite, 1903), chap. 1.

10   Pierre Janet, *Les Obsessions et la psychasthenie,* 2 vols. (Paris: Félix Alcan, 1903), 2: 356–73.

11   Eugenio Tanzi, *A Text-Book of Mental Diseases,* trans. W. Ford Robertson and T. C. Mackenzie (New York: Rebman, 1910).

12   *La psicanalisi: Studii ed appunti critici,* 2 vols. (Turin: Bocca, 1926). See also Morselli's essay "La psicologia etnica e la scienza eugenistica," *International Eugenics Congress—1912,* 2 vols. (London: Eugenics Education Society, 1912), 1: 58–62. On Morselli, see Patrizia Guanieri, *Individualit à difformi: La psichiatria antropologica di Enrico Morselli* (Milan: F. Angeli, 1986).

13   Edoardo Weiss, *Sigmund Freud as a Consultant: Reflections of a Pioneer in Psychoanalysis* (New York: International Medical Book Corporation, 1970), pp. 51–55.

14   Sigmund Freud, *Briefe 1873-1939,* ed., Ernst Freud and Lucie Freud (Frankfurt/M.: Fischer, 1960), p. 380.

15   Wilhelm Stekel, *Compulsion and Doubt,* trans. Emil A. Gutheil, 2 vols. (New York: Liveright, 1949), 1: 131. All quotations are from this edition. The book was originally published as *Zwang und Zweifel, für Ärzte und Mediziner dargestellt,* 2 vols. (Berlin: Urban und Schwarzenberg, 1927).

16   Jacques Joseph, *Rhinoplasty and Facial Plastic Surgery with a Supplement on Mammaplasty and Other Operations in the Field of Plastic Surgery of the Body,* trans. Stanley Milstein (Phoenix: Columella Press, 1987), p. 743. All quotations are from this edition. The book was originally published as *Nasenplastik und sonstige Gesichtsplastik, nebst einem Anhang über Mammaplastik und einige weitere Operationen aus dem Gebiete der äusseren Körperplastik: Ein Atlas und ein Lehrbuch* (Leipzig: C. Kabitzsch, 1931).

17   Walter Jahrreis, "Das hypochrondrische Denken," *Archiv für Psychiatrie und Nervenkrankheiten* 92 (1930): 686–823.

18   Heinrich Stutte, "Thersites-Komplex," *A criança portuguesa* 21 (1962–1963): 451–56, and Stutte et al., eds., *Ergebnisse und Probleme der Sozialpsychiatrie* (Stuttgart: H. Huber, 1958).

19   Heinz Dietrich, "Über Dysmorphie (Mißgestaltfurcht)," *Archiv für Psychiatrie und Nervenkrankheiten* 203 (1962): 511–18.

20   Berndorfer, "Aesthetic Surgery as Organopsychic Therapy," pp. 144–45.

21   R. G. Druss, F. C. Symonds, and G. F. Crikelair, "The Problem of So-

matic Delusions in Patients Seeking Cosmetic Surgery," *Plastic and Reconstructive Surgery* 48 (1971): 246–50.

22 Bettman, p. 184.

23 Natvig, *Jacques Joseph: Surgical Sculptor* pp. 23–24. See also the other sources on Joseph cited above, p. 171 n. 5.

24 Edmund Saalfeld, *Lectures on Cosmetic Treatment: A Manual for Practitioners*, trans., J. F. Halls Dally (London: Rebman, 1911), pp. 106–7.

25 Bernard H. Shulman, "Psychiatric Assessment of the Candidate for Cosmetic Surgery," *Otolyryngologic Clinics of North America* 13 (1980): 389.

26 Hiroyuki Ohjimi, Nobuyuki Shioya, and Jun Ishigooka, "The Role of Psychiatry in Aesthetic Surgery," *Aesthetic Plastic Surgery* 12 (1988): 187–90.

27 P. Clarkson and D. Stafford-Clark, "The Relationship of Appearance to Mental Health," in A. B. Wallace, ed., *Transactions of the International Society of Plastic Surgeons, Second Congress* (Edinburgh: E. and S. Livingstone, 1960), pp. 492–95.

28 The *Diagnostic and Statistical Manual of Mental Disorders* (Washington, DC: American Psychiatric Association, 1952; 2d ed., 1968; 3d ed., 1980; 3d ed., rev., 1987; 4th ed., 1994) is the standard American (and in general now global) guide to diagnostic criteria for mental illness. On DSM-III and aesthetic surgery, see Louis Linn, "Cosmetic Surgery, with Particular Reference to Rhinoplasty," in Richard S. Blacher, ed., *The Psychological Experience of Surgery* (New York: John Wiley and Sons, 1987), pp. 194–206.

29 N. C. Andreasen and J. Bardach, "Dysmorphophobia: Symptom or Disease?" *American Journal of Psychiatry* 134 (1977): 673–76.

30 Katharine A. Phillips, "An Open Study of Buspirone Augmentation of Serotonin-Reuptake Inhibitors in Body Dysmorphic Disorder," *Psychopharmacology Bulletin* 32 (1996): 175–80. See also Eric Hollander et al., "Body Dysmorphic Disorder: Diagnostic Issues and Related Disorders," *Psychosomatics* 33 (1992): 156–65.

31 See Katharine A. Phillips et al., "Body Dysmorphic Disorder: An Obsessive-Compulsive Spectrum Disorder, a Form of Affective Spectrum Disorder, or Both?" *Journal of Clinical Psychiatry* 56, Supplement 4 (1995): 41–51, discussion, 52; and S. L. McElroy et al., "Body Dysmorphic Disorder: Does It Have a Psychotic Subtype?" *Journal of Clinical Psychiatry* 54 (1993): 389–95.

32 "Baldies and Jackson, Beware BDD Bogey—Psychiatrist," Reuters World Service, (July 10, 1996): BC cycle.

33 See the discussion throughout John Money and Herman Musaph, eds.,

The Handbook of Sexology (Amsterdam: Excerpta medica, 1977), for example, pp. 171, 487, 1295, 1309.

3. ERNST KRETSCHMER'S CONSTITUTIONAL NOSES

1   Moses Hess, Rom und Jerusalem, 2d ed. (Leipzig: M. W. Kaufmann, 1899), Brief IV. Cited in the translation from Paul Lawrence Rose, Revolutionary Antisemitism in Germany from Kant to Wagner (Princeton: Princeton University Press, 1990), p. 323.

2   All references to the text are to Thomas Mann, "The Blood of the Walsungs," in Death in Venice and Seven Other Stories, trans. H. T. Lowe-Porter (New York: Vintage, 1989), pp. 289–316. This translates the "official" version of the story without the Yiddish ending. The German text in the complete edition is the same text: Thomas Mann, Frühe Erzählungen (Frankfurt/M.: S. Fischer, 1981), pp. 493–524.

3   All of these references are from a single page (26) in Hans F. K. Günther, Rassenkunde des jüdischen Volkes (1922; repr., Munich: J. F. Lehmann, 1930).

4   Eden Warwick, Notes on Noses (1848; repr., London: Richard Bentley, 1864), p. 11. On the general question of the representation of the physiognomy of the Jew in mid-nineteenth-century culture, see Mary Cowling, The Artist as Anthropologist: The Representation of Type and Character in Victorian Art (Cambridge: Cambridge University Press, 1989), pp. 118–19, 332–33.

5   Bernhard Blechmann, Ein Beitrag zur Anthropologie der Juden (Dorpat: Wilhelm Just, 1882), p. 11.

6   Joseph Jacobs, Studies in Jewish Statistics, Social, Vital and Anthropometric (London: D. Nutt, 1891), p. xxxii.

7   John R. Baker, Race (New York: Oxford University Press, 1974), p. 241.

8   Hans Leicher, Die Vererbung anatomischer Variationen der Nase: Ihrer Nebenhöhlen und des Gehörorgans (Munich: J. F. Bergmann, 1928), pp. 80–85.

9   Roland Barthes, Camera Lucida, trans. Richard Howard (New York: Hill and Wang, 1981), p. 105.

10   Moysheh Oyved, Gems and Life (London: Ernest Benn, 1927), p. 71.

11   William Saroyan, The Human Comedy (New York, 1943), p. 63.

12   Cited from an interview by Neal Gabler, An Empire of Their Own: How the Jews Invented Hollywood (New York: Crown, 1988), pp. 242–43.

13   Julian Barnes, Metroland (London: Jonathan Cape: 1980), p. 32.

14   See the discussion in Hyman L. Muslin, "The Jew in Literature: The

Hated Self," *Israel Journal of Psychiatry and Related Science* 27 (1990): 1–16.

15   Ronald Steel, *Walter Lippmann and the American Century* (Boston: Little, Brown, 1980), p. 192.

16   Ernst Kretschmer, *Körperbau und Charakter: Untersuchungen zum Konstitutionsproblem und zur Lehre von den Temperamenten* (Berlin: Springer, 1922). The best presentation of the debates between the racialist and nonracialist readings of constitution theory remains William Armand Lessa, *Landmarks in the Science of Human Types* ([New York:] Brooklyn College Press, 1942).

17   Ludwig Stern-Piper, "Zur Frage der Bedeutung der psycho-physischen Typen," *Zeitschrift für die gesamte Neurologie und Psychiatrie* 84 (1923): 408–14.

18   Ernst Kretschmer, "Konstitution und Rasse," *Zeitschrift für die gesamte Neurologie und Psychiatrie* 82 (1923): 139–47. One should note that Kretschmer was refused a chair in psychiatry at Tübingen in January 1945 because of his "political worldview," that is, because of his refusal to accept the arguments of racial science. See the letter of Stickl, the Rector of the University of Tübingen in Kretschmer's "Personalnotizen" (1945) from "Der Bevollmächtigte für das Sanitäts- und Gesundheitswesen" at the Berlin Documentation Center.

19   Ludwig Stern-Piper, "Konstitution und Rasse," *Zeitschrift für die gesamte Neurologie und Psychiatrie* 86 (1923): 265–73.

20   M. J. Gutmann, "Geisteskrankheiten bei Juden," *Zeitschrift für Demographie und Statistik der Juden*, n.s. 3 (1926): 109.

21   Julius Tandler, "Konstitution und Rassenhygiene," *Zeitschrift für angewandte Anatomie und Konstitutionslehre* 1 (1914): 11–26.

22   Werner Sombart, *The Jews and Modern Capitalism*, trans. M. Epstein (Glencoe, Ill.: Free Press, 1951), pp. 271–72.

23   "Kultur des Geistes," *Kulturmensch* (October 15, 1904): 19–20.

24   "Types," *The Jewish Encyclopedia*, 12 vols. (New York: Funk and Wagnalls, 1906), 12: 295. On this general argument, see John M. Efron, *Defenders of the Race: Jewish Doctors and Race Science in Fin-de-siècle Europe* (New Haven: Yale University Press, 1994).

25   Heinrich Heine, *Werke*, ed. Klaus Briegleb, 12 vols. (Berlin: Ullstein, 1981), 7: 31.

26   Wilhelm Busch, *Gesamtausgabe*, ed. Friedrich Bohne, 4 vols. (Wiesbaden: Emil Vollmer, [n.d.]): 2: 204; the English translation, which is very accurate to the tone, but not to the order of the parts of the Jew's body, is from Walter Arndt, comp. and trans., *The Genius of Wilhelm Busch* (Berkeley: University of California Press, 1982), p. 42.

27 Compare Alfred Berndorfer, *Die Aesthetik der Nase: Vom plastisch-chirurgischen Standpunkt aus betrachtet* (Vienna: Wilhelm Maudrich, 1949).

28 Berndorfer, "Aesthetic Surgery as Organopsychic Therapy," p. 143.

29 Hans Blüher, *Secessio Judaica: Philosophische Grundlegung der historischen Situation des Judenthums und der antisemitischen Bewegung* (Berlin: Der weisse Ritter, 1922), p. 23. On Blüher's extraordinary impact on Jewish thinkers of the time, see Alex Bein's autobiographical footnote on Blüher in Alex Bein, "The Jewish Parasite," *Leo Baeck Yearbook* 9 (1964): 14 n. 39.

4. SIGMUND FREUD'S NOSE JOB

1 See Sander L. Gilman, *Disease and Representation: Images of Illness from Madness to AIDS* (Ithaca, N.Y.: Cornell University Press, 1988), pp. 182–201.

2 Frank J. Sulloway, *Freud, Biologist of the Mind: Beyond the Psychoanalytic Legend* (New York: Basic Books, 1983), pp. 152, 148–50.

3 "The Relation between the Nose and the Sexual Apparatus," *Boston Medical and Surgical Journal* 138 (1898): 139.

4 Wilhelm Fliess, *Die Beziehungen zwischen Nase und weiblichen Geschlechtsorganen: In ihrer biologischen Bedeutung dargestellt* (Leipzig: Franz Deuticke, 1897).

5 On the symbolic value of this manifestation see Herbert Ian Hogbin, *The Island of Menstruating Men; Religion in Wogeo, New Guinea* (Scranton, Pa.: Chandler, 1970), and James L. Brain, "Male Menstruation in History and Anthropology," *Journal of Psychohistory* 15 (1988): 311–23.

6 *The Complete Letters of Sigmund Freud to Wilhelm Fliess, 1887–1904*, ed. Jeffrey Moussaieff Masson (Cambridge, Mass.: Harvard University Press, 1985), p. 256.

7 Freud, *Complete Letters . . . to Fliess*, p. 270.

8 See, for example, F. A. Forel, "Cas de menstruation chez un homme," *Bulletin de la Société médicale de la Suisse romande* (Lausanne), 1869, 53–61, and W. D. Halliburton, "A Peculiar Case," *Weekly Medical Review and Journal of Obstetrics* (St. Louis), 1885, 392.

9 Paolo Albrecht, "Sulla mestruazione ne maschio," *L'Anomalo* 2 (1980): 33.

10 Paul Näcke, "Kritisches zum Kapitel der normalen und pathologischen Sexualität," *Archiv für Psychiatrie und Nervenkrankheiten* 32 (1899): 364–65. On Freud and Näcke, see Helmut Gröger, "Sigmund Freud an

Paul Näcke, Erstveröffentlichung zweier Freud-Briefe," *Luzifer Amor* 3 (1990): 144–62.

11 Magnus Hirschfeld, *Sexualpathologie*, 2 vols. (Bonn: A. Marcus und E. Weber, 1917–1918), 2: 1–92.

12 Freud, *Complete Letters . . . to Fliess*, p. 272. Compare the rather spare discussion in Peter Gay, *Freud: A Life for Our Times* (New York: Norton, 1988), pp. 84–86.

13 Leopold Schönbauer, *Das medizinische Wien* (Berlin, Vienna: Urban and Schwarzenberg, 1944), p. 294.

14 A. Fraenkel, "Robert Gersuny," *Deutsche Medizinische Wochenschrift* 50 (1924): 2.

15 Robert Gersuny, *Doctors and Patients: Hints to Both*, trans. A. S. Levetus (Bristol: John Wright, 1898).

16 Moriz Weil, "Zur Pathologie und Therapie der Eiterungen der Nasennebenhöhlen," *Wiener medizinische Wochenschrift* 47 (1897): 706–10, 761–65, 814–19, 909–13, 965–68, cited in Masson, p. 216.

17 SE 20: 233.

18 "Nase," *Handwörterbuch des deutschen Aberglaubens*, 10 vols., ed. Hanns Bächtold-Stäubli (Berlin and Leipzig: Walter de Gruyter, 1934–1935), 6: 970–79; and Havelock Ellis, *Sexual Selection in Man*, vol. 4 of *Studies in the Psychology of Sex* (Philadelphia: F. A. Davis, 1905), pp. 67–69.

19 On this principle of reversal and the meaning of the nose as a symbol of the castrated penis, see Otto Fenichel, "Die 'lange Nase,' " *Imago* 14 (1928): 502–4.

20 See Jay Geller, "The Aromatics of Jewish Difference; or, Benjamin's Allegory of Aura," in Jonathan Boyarin and Daniel Boyarin, eds., *Jews and Other Differences: The New Jewish Cultural Studies* (Minneapolis: University of Minnesota Press, 1997), pp. 203–56.

21 John Grand-Carteret, *L'Affaire Dreyfus et l'image* (Paris: E. Flammarion, 1898); Eduard Fuchs, *Die Juden in der Karikatur* (Munich: Langen, 1921); and Judith Vogt, *Historien om et Image: Antisemitisme og Antizionisme i Karikaturer* (Copenhagen: Samieren, 1978).

22 See Dietz Bering, *Der Name als Stigma: Antisemitismus im deutschen Alltag 1812–1933* (Stuttgart: Klett/Cotta, 1987), p. 211.

23 Friedrich Nietzsche, *Beyond Good and Evil*, trans. Marianne Cowan (Chicago: Henry Regnery, 1955), pp. 184–88.

24 Oskar Hovorka, *Die äussere Nase: Eine anatomisch-anthropologische Studie* (Vienna: Alfred Hölder, 1893), pp. 130–40. On the pathological meaning of the nose in German science for the later period, see Leicher, p. 81.

25 Arthur Landsberger, ed., *Judentaufe* (Munich: Georg Müller, 1912), p. 45.

5. SIGMUND FREUD'S CASTRATION ANXIETY

1 See Sander L. Gilman, *Jewish Self-Hatred: Anti-Semitism and the Hidden Language of the Jews* (Baltimore: Johns Hopkins University Press, 1986), pp. 193–94.

2 *Minutes of the Vienna Psychoanalytic Society*, trans. M. Nunberg, 4 vols. (New York: International Universities Press, 1962–1975), 2: 73–74. The minutes were originally published as *Protokolle der Wiener Psychoanalytischen Vereinigung*, ed. Herman Nunberg and Ernst Federn, 4 vols. (Frankfurt a. M.: Fischer, 1976–1981), 1: 66–67.

3 SE 10: 36.

4 SE 10: 36. On the meaning given circumcision and its relationship to anti-Semitism within the psychoanalytic tradition, see Georges Maranz, "Les Conséquences de la circoncision: Essai d'explication psychanalytique de l'antisémitisme," *Psyché-Paris* 2 (1947): 731–45; B. Grunberger, "Circoncision et l'antisémitisme: En marge d'un article de Georges Maranz," *Psyché-Paris* 2 (1947): 1221–28; Jules Glenn, "Circumcision and Anti-Semitism," *Psychoanalytic Quarterly* 29 (1960): 395–99.

5 Max Graf, "Reminiscences of Professor Sigmund Freud," *Psychoanalytic Quarterly* 11 (1942): 473.

6 SE 17: 86.

7 SE 17: 86.

8 Ruth Mack Brunswick, "A Supplement to Freud's 'History of an Infantile Neurosis,'" *International Journal of Psychoanalysis* 9 (1928): 439–76.

6. ALFRED ADLER'S INFERIORITY COMPLEX

1 On the history of this concept, see Oliver Brachfeld, *Inferiority Feelings in the Individual and the Group*, trans. Marjorie Gabain (Westport, Conn.: Greenwood, 1972).

2 Haiken, "Body and Soul: Plastic Surgery in the United States, 1914–1990," pp. 191–245.

3 Alfred Adler, *Study of Organ Inferiority and Its Psychical Compensation: A Contribution to Clinical Medicine*, trans. Smith Ely Jelliffe (New York: Nervous and Mental Disease Publishing Company, 1917). Adler's study was originally published as *Studie über Minder-*

wertigkeit von Organen (Berlin: Urban und Schwarzenberg, 1907). See Edward Hoffman, *The Drive for Self: Alfred Adler and the Founding of Individual Psychology* (Reading, MA: Addison-Wesley, 1994); Hannes Bohringer, *Kompensation und Common Sense: Zur Lebensphilosophie Alfred Adlers* (Königstein: Hain Verlag bei Athenaum, 1985); Paul E. Stepansky, *Adler in Context* (Hillside, NJ: Analytic Press, 1983); Henry Jacoby, *Alfred Adlers Individualpsychologie und dialektische Charakterkunde* (Frankfurt a. M.: Fischer-Taschenbuch, 1974); Almuth Bruder-Bezzel, *Alfred Adler: Die Entstehungsgeschichte einer Theorie im historischen Milieu Wiens* (Göttingen: Vandenhoeck und Ruprecht, 1983).

4 The best and most detailed study of the German reception is Mariacarla Gadebusch Bondio, *Die Rezeption der kriminalanthropologischen Theorien von Cesare Lombroso in Deutschland von 1800–1914* (Hüsum: Matthiesen, 1995). In general see also Robert A. Nye, "Heredity or Milieu: The Foundations of Modern European Criminological Theory," *Isis* 67 (1976): 335–55.

5 Kraepelin, *Psychiatrie*, 2: 331–37. On Kraepelin's ideological background, see Eric J. Engstrom, "Emil Kraepelin: Psychiatry and Public Affairs in Wilhelmine Germany," *History of Psychiatry* 2 (1991): 111–32.

6 Julius Friedrich Cohnheim, *Die Tuberkulose vom Standpunkte der Infectionslehre* (Leipzig: A. Edelmann, 1880), p. 34.

7 *Minutes of the Vienna Psychoanalytic Society*, 1: 43.

8 Erwin Baur, Eugen Fischer, and Fritz Lenz, *Menschliche Erblichkeitslehre und Rassenhygiene*, 3 vols. (München: J. F. Lehmann, 1921), 1: 213.

9 Baur, Fischer, and Lenz, 1: 20–21.

10 Alfred Adler, *The Neurotic Constitution: Outlines of a Comparative Individualistic Psychology and Psychotherapy*, trans. Bernard Glueck and John E. Lind (New York: Moffat, Yard, 1917). Adler's original text was published as *Über den nervosen Charakter: Grundzüge einer vergleichenden Individual-Psychologie und Psychotherapie* (Wiesbaden: J. F. Bergmann, 1912). By 1928 it was in its fourth German edition.

11 Adler, *The Neurotic Constitution*, p. 27.

12 Maxwell Maltz, *New Faces, New Futures: Rebuilding Character with Plastic Surgery* (New York: Richard R. Smith, 1936), p. ix.

13 Maxwell Maltz, *Doctor Pygmalion: The Autobiography of a Plastic Surgeon* (New York: Thomas J. Crowell, 1953), pp. 5–6.

14 Vilray P. Blair, "Operations for Relief of Hare Lip and Cleft Palate," *Hygeia* 4 (1926): 325–26.

15 William Wesley Carter, "The Importance of Nasal Plastic Surgery," *Laryngoscope* 40 (1930): 502.

16 Clarence R. Straatsma, "Plastic Surgery: Its Uses and Limitations," *New York Journal of Medicine* 32 (March 1, 1932): 254.

17 Charles R. Stockard, *The Physical Basis of Personality* (New York: Norton, 1931), p. 215.

18 William E. Carter, "Physical Findings in Problem Children," *Mental Hygiene* 10 (1926): 75–84.

19 Lawson G. Lowry, "Competitions and the Conflict over Difference: The Inferiority Complex in the Psychopathology of Childhood," *Mental Hygiene* 12 (1928): 316–30.

20 Walter de la Mare, *Broomsticks and Other Tales* (New York: Knopf, 1925), pp. 175–226.

21 Robert M. Goldwyn, "The Paraffin Story," *Plastic and Reconstructive Surgery* 65 (1980): 517–24.

7. PAUL SCHILDER'S SOCIAL BODY

1 Bettman, "The Psychology of Appearances," p. 182.

2 Gillies, *The Development and Scope of Plastic Surgery*, pp. 26, 31.

3 Gillies and Millard, 2: 320.

4 Jacques W. Maliniak, "American Society of Plastic and Reconstructive Surgery: Its Beginning, Objectives, and Progress, 1932–1947," *Plastic and Reconstructive Surgery* 2 (1947): 518.

5 Paul Schilder, *The Image and Appearance of the Human Body: Studies in the Constructive Energies of the Psyche* (London: K. Paul, Trench, Trubner, 1935). This is a much expanded and rethought version of his *Das Körperschema: Ein Beitrag zur Lehre vom Bewusstsein des eigenen Körpers* (Berlin: Springer, 1923).

6 On the distinctions among the various constructions of the body, see John O'Neill, *Five Bodies: The Human Shape of Modern Society* (Ithaca, N.Y.: Cornell University Press, 1985). On the social body, see pp. 48–66.

7 Eric L. Santner, *My Own Private Germany: Daniel Paul Schreber's Secret History of Modernity* (Princeton, N.J.: Princeton University Press, 1996).

8. KARL MENNINGER'S POLYSURGERY

1 See the most recent extensive study by Margaret Louise Sartori, "Patient Dissatisfaction and Elective Cosmetic Surgery: An Empirical Study" (diss., University of Detroit, 1992).

2 Karl A. Menninger, "Polysurgery and Polysurgical Addiction," *Psychoanalytic Quarterly* 3 (1934): 173–99.

3 Ernest Hemingway, *The Sun Also Rises* (New York: Charles Scribner's

Sons, 1954), p. 4. See Michael S. Reynolds, *"The Sun Also Rises": A Novel of the Twenties* (Boston: Twayne, 1995).

4 Helene Deutsch, "Some Psychoanalytic Observations in Surgery," *Psychosomatic Medicine* 4 (1942): 105–15.

5 On Deutsch and the question of male circumcision, see Sander L. Gilman, "Salome, Syphilis, Sarah Bernhardt, and the Modern Jewess," in Linda Nochlin and Tamar Garb, eds., *The Jew in the Text* (London: Thames and Hudson, 1995), pp. 119–21.

6 Erich Lindemann, "Observations on Psychiatric Sequelae to Surgical Operations in Women," *American Journal of Psychiatry* 98 (1941): 132–39.

7 Certainly the best overview of Talcott Parsons's representation of illness and the patient remains Bryan S. Turner, "Sickness and Social Structure: Parsons's Contribution to Medical Sociology," in Robert J. Holton and Bryan S. Turner, eds., *Talcott Parsons on Economy and Society* (London: Routledge, 1986), pp. 107–42. See Talcott Parsons and Renée Fox, *Illness, Therapy and the Modern Urban American Family* (Indianapolis, Ind.: Bobbs-Merrill, 1967).

8 Phyllis Greenacre, "Surgical Addiction—A Case Illustration," *Psychosomatic Medicine* 1 (1939): 325–28.

9 Knorr, Edgerton, and Hoopes, pp. 285–89.

10 Vilray Papin Blair and James Barrett Brown, "Nasal Abnormalities, Fancied and Real: The Reaction of the Patient: Their Attempted Correction," *Surgery, Gynecology, Obstetrics* 53 (1931): 797–819.

9. GOD'S AESTHETIC SURGERY

1 Julius Preuss, *Biblisch-talmudische Medizin: Beiträge zur Geschichte der Heilkunde und der Kultur überhaupt* (Berlin: S. Karger, 1911), pp. 339–41.

2 Fred Rosner and J. David Bleich, eds., *Jewish Bioethics* (New York: Sanhedrin Press, 1979); J. David Bleich, *Contemporary Halakhic Problems*, 4 vols. (New York: Ktav, 1977–1995).

3 Lawrence A. Hoffman, *Covenant of Blood: Circumcision and Gender in Rabbinic Judaism* (Chicago: University of Chicago Press, 1996).

4 Adolf Jellinek, *Der Jüdische Stamm* (Wien: Herzfeld und Bauer, 1869), pp. 44–45.

5 A sense of how very different the attitude toward aesthetic surgery is among younger Jews in the United Kingdom today can be found in the recent piece by Ruth Getz, "Drastic Surgery" in the hip new magazine for Jewish generation Xers, *New Moon/Not Quite Kosher* (September 1997): 12–18.

6 See J. David Bleich, *Judaism and Healing: Halakhic Perspectives* (New York: KTAV, 1981), pp. 126–28.

7 See, for example, Rogers, "A Brief History of Cosmetic Surgery," as well as Rogers, "A Chronological History of Cosmetic Surgery."

8 Bleich, *Judaism and Healing*, 127.

9 Charles G. O'Leary, "Catholic Views on Cosmetic Surgery," *Eye, Ear, Nose, and Throat Monthly* 41 (1962): 60.

10 Quoted by Joseph G. McCarthy, "Introduction to Plastic Surgery," in *General Principles*, vol. 1 of *Plastic Surgery*, 8 vols. (Philadelphia: W. B. Saunders, 1990), p. 24.

10. PRESCOTT LECKY'S SELF-CONSISTENCY

1 See Goldwyn, *The Patient and the Plastic Surgeon*, pp. 9–51; V. Micheli-Pellegrini and G. M. Manfrida, "Rhinoplasty and Its Psychological Implications: Applied Psychological Observations in Aesthetic Surgery," *Aesthetic Plastic Surgery* 3 (1979): 299–319; Mary Kay Coco, "Psychosocial Aspects of Physical Appearance: A Study in Aesthetic Surgery" (diss., University of Utah, 1980); and Ellen Ribner, "Pre-operative Patient Attitudes and Surgical Outcome: A Pilot Study of Elective Nasal Patients" (diss., San Jose State University, 1990).

2 Bruce J. Crispin et al., *Contemporary Esthetic Dentistry: Practice Fundamentals* (Tokyo: Quintessence, 1994), p. 11.

3 Jeffrey D. Robertson and William T. Keavy, *Plastic Surgery: Malpractice and Damages* (New York: Wiley Law Publications, 1990); *Medical Malpractice: Handling Plastic Surgery Cases*, ed. Robert L. Cucin (Colorado Springs, CO: Shepard's/McGraw-Hill; New York: McGraw-Hill, 1990).

4 Charles Conrad Miller, *Cosmetic Surgery: The Correction of Featural Imperfections* (Philadelphia: F.A. Davis, 1924), p. 255. See Haiken, "Body and Soul," pp. 39–45.

5 Wengle, pp. 435–43.

6 M. R. Wright and W. K. Wright, "A Psychological Study of Patients Undergoing Cosmetic Surgery," *Archive of Otolaryngology* 101 (1975): 145–51.

7 Sartori.

8 M. T. Edgerton, W. E. Jacobson, and E. Meyer, "Surgical-Psychiatric Study of Patients Seeking Plastic (Cosmetic) Surgery: Ninety-eight Consecutive Patients with Minimal Deformity," *British Journal of Plastic Surgery* 13 (1961): 136–45; M. T. Edgerton and N. J. Knorr, "Motivational Patterns of Patients Seeking Cosmetic (Esthetic) Surgery," *Plastic and Reconstructive Surgery* 48 (1971): 551–57; M. T. Edgerton et al., "Psychi-

atric Evaluation of Male Patients Seeking Cosmetic Surgery," *Plastic and Reconstructive Surgery* 26 (1960): 356–72; M. T. Edgerton, W. E. Jacobson, and E. Meyer, "Psychiatric Contributions to the Clinical Management of Plastic-Surgery Patients," *Postgraduate Medicine* 29 (1961): 513–21; M. T. Edgerton, W. E. Jacobson, and E. Meyer, "Motivational Patterns in Patients Seeking Elective Plastic Surgery: I. Women Who Seek Rhinoplasty," *Psychosomatic Medicine* 22 (1960): 193–201; W. L. Webb Jr., et al., "Mechanisms of Psychosocial Adjustment in Patients Seeking 'Face-Lift' Operations," *Psychosomatic Medicine* 27 (1965): 183–92.

9   Louis Linn and Irving B. Goldman, "Psychiatric Observations Concerning Rhinoplasty," *Psychosomatic Medicine* 11 (1949): 307–14.

10   Frances Cooke Macgregor, *Transformation and Identity: The Face and Plastic Surgery* (New York: Quadrangle Press, 1974), p. 2.

11   Frances Cooke Macgregor and Bertram Schaffner, "Screening Patients for Nasal Plastic Operations," *Psychosomatic Medicine* 12 (1950): 283–84.

12   Goin and Goin, p. 133.

13   The literature on the psychology of the rhinoplasty patient is both extensive and not very rich. Recent exceptions that are informative and thought-provoking are Sarah Moses, Uriel Last, and Dan Mahler, "Mental Health Correlates of Valid Perception of Nasal Deformity in Female Applicants for Aesthetic Surgery," *Aesthetic Plastic Surgery* 7 (1983): 77–80; Sarah Moses, Uriel Last, and Dan Mahler, "After Aesthetic Rhinoplasty: New Looks and Psychological Outlooks on Postsurgical Satisfaction," *Aesthetic Plastic Surgery* 8 (1984): 213–17; Jean Ann Graham and Albert M. Kligman, eds., *The Psychology of Cosmetic Treatments* (New York: Praeger, 1985); Lennart Meyer and Sten Jacobsen, "Psychiatric and Psychosocial Characteristics of Patients Accepted for Rhinoplasty," *Annals of Plastic Surgery* 19 (1987): 117–30; A. A. Robin et al., "Reshaping the Psyche: The Concurrent Improvement in Appearance and Mental State after Rhinoplasty," *British Journal of Psychiatry* 152 (1988): 539–43; Mary Ruth Wright, "The Psychology of Rhinoplasty," *Facial Plastic Surgery* 5 (1988): 109–13; R. Feiss and J. P. Real, "Rhinoplastie: Aspects psychiques: Collaboration Psychiatre/Chirurgien," *Annales de chirugie plastique et esthétique* 34 (1989): 392–94.

14   Julien Reich, "The Interface of Plastic Surgery and Psychiatry," *Clinics in Plastic Surgery* 9 (1982): 372.

15   Leon Festinger, *A Theory of Cognitive Dissonance* (Stanford, Calif.: Stanford University Press, 1965).

16 Prescott Lecky, *Self-Consistency: A Theory of Personality* (Fort Myers Beach, Fla.: Island Press, 1982).

17 Victor Charles Raimy, *The Self-Concept As a Factor in Counseling and Personality Organization* (Columbus: Office of Educational Services, Ohio State University Libraries, 1971), p. 121.

18 Judith Burke, Seymour L. Zelen, and Edward O. Terino, "More than Skin Deep: A Self-Consistency Approach to the Psychology of Cosmetic Surgery," *Plastic and Reconstructive Surgery* 76 (1985): 270.

19 Marsha L. Richins, "Social Comparison and the Idealized Images of Advertising," *Journal of Consumer Research* 18 (1991): 71.

20 Donald Snygg and A. W. Combs, *Individual Behavior: A New Frame of Reference for Psychology* (New York: Harper, 1949), pp. 99–100.

21 R. M. Bittle, "Psychiatric Evaluation of Patients Seeking Rhinoplasty," *Otolaryngologic Clinics of North America* 8 (1975): 689–704.

22 Davis.

23 Burk, Zelen, and Terino, pp. 270–80.

24 Susan C. Shore, "An Exploratory Study of Postoperative Trauma and Depression among Cosmetic Surgery Recipients" (diss., Union Institute, 1992).

25 Gifford.

26 J. G. Stafne, "The Cosmetic Surgery Patient: Why Do They Do It to Themselves?" *Minnesota Medicine* 63 (1980): 175–77, 209.

Index

Sander L. Gilman is Henry R. Luce Professor of
the Liberal Arts in Human Biology and chair of the
Department of Germanic Studies at the University of
Chicago. He is the author of *Smart Jews: The Construction of the Image of Jewish Superior Intelligence*
and *Picturing Health and Illness: Images of Identity
and Difference*, as well as numerous other books.

Library of Congress Cataloging-in-Publication Data
Gilman, Sander L.
Creating beauty to cure the soul : race and psychology
in the shaping of aesthetic surgery / Sander L. Gilman.
Includes index.
ISBN 0-8223-2111-4 (hardcover : alk. paper).
ISBN 0-8223-2144-0 (pbk. : alk. paper)
1. Surgery, Plastic—Psychological aspects.   2. Beauty,
Personal—Psychological aspects.   3. Surgery, Plastic—
Philosophy.   I. Title.
RD118.5.G55   1998   617.9′5′019—dc21   98-23182 CIP